Copyright © 2026 by Jermaine Jefferson
All rights reserved.

The author or publisher does not permit reproducing, storing in a retrieval system, or transmitting any part of this book in any form or by any means, electronic, mechanical, photocopying, recording, or otherwise, without prior written permission, except as permitted under United States copyright law.

First edition ISBN 9798297544123
Second edition ISBN 9798994773222

Published by GrowFitFL Publishing
Printed in the United States of America

The author provides this book for informational and educational purposes only. The author is not a licensed professional; therefore, you should not interpret this book's content as medical, legal, or professional advice. Readers must fully assume responsibility for how they use the information in this book.

All trademarks, product names, and company names mentioned are the property of their respective owners. Their use does not imply endorsement.

Contents

Title Page	VII
Thank You	1
Dedication	3
Prologue	5
Introduction	8
1. Chapter 1 Not Built For Us	10
2. Chapter 2 The Hidden Cost	19
3. Chapter 3 Your Health Is a Garden	25
4. Chapter 4 Nobody's Coming to Save You	37
5. Chapter 5 Start Where You Are	48
6. Chapter 6 Year Round Garden	59

7. Chapter 7 — 104
   Medicinal Herbs

8. Chapter 8 — 137
   Time & Money

9. Chapter 9 — 154
   Why I Train Like I Grow

10. Chapter 10 — 171
    The Home Trilogy

11. Chapter 11 — 184
    Mental Health

12. Chapter 12 — 197
    Raising Healthy Kids

13. Chapter 13 — 209
    Planting Trees You'll Never Climb

14. Chapter 14 — 219
    The Florida Survivor Fifteen

15. Chapter 15 — 242
    Everyday Warrior

16. Chapter 16 — 252
    Side Hustle Roots

17. Chapter 17 — 261
    The Garden After You

18. Chapter 18 — 264
    The Call To Action

19.	Chapter 19 Winter Protection	270
20.	Chapter 20 Recovery after Disaster	279
21.	Chapter 21 Why do I grow?	287

Closing Words	290
Author's Note	
About The Author	292
Acknowledgments	294
In Loving Memory of My Father	296

Grow Food Not Lawns Copy

Simple Steps To Turn Any Yard Into A Year-Round Garden

Jermaine Jefferson

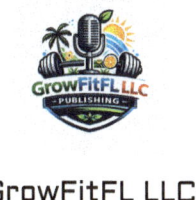

GrowFitFL LLC

Thank You

Thank you for choosing this book.

In a world full of shortcuts, noise, and distractions, you made a deliberate decision to slow down and learn something that actually matters. Growing food. Building resilience. Creating a healthier life for yourself and the people you care about. That choice alone says a lot about you.

Everything on these pages comes from experience. Successes, mistakes, setbacks, and seasons where nothing went according to plan. I am not writing from theory or trends. I am writing from years of doing this in real Florida soil, under actual heat, storms, and pressure, while raising a family and figuring things out as I go.

If this book resonates with you, there is more.

I share ongoing lessons, practical demonstrations, and real-life updates on my YouTube channel, GrowFitFL, where you can see these ideas applied day by day in our backyard. It extends this book, not polished perfection, just honest work and steady progress.

You can also learn more about my background, current projects, and the bigger mission behind this work at jermainejefferson.com. That site connects everything I am building, writing, and teaching in one place.

I hope this book does more than inform you. I hope it encourages you. Ground you. Reminds you that growing food, improving your health, and taking responsibility for your environment is not extreme. It is human.

Thank you for being here, for reading, and for choosing to grow.

Dedication

2025 has been the most challenging year of my life.

Losing my dad still doesn't feel real. It's hard to fathom that I'm living in a world where my father is no longer physically present.

This is the man from whom I used to seek advice. The one who made flying home feels like home. The one who gave the biggest hugs and asked for nothing more than time with his family. His absence isn't just felt by me; it's shaken our entire family.

He was the leader. The general. The one who always knew what to say and what to do. My dad is the reason I started GrowFitFL, which has quickly become one of the fastest-growing gardening and health channels on YouTube. He told me, "You've got so much knowledge in this space; maybe it's God's plan for you to share it and help others live healthier, happier lives."

That seed he planted in me is what grew into this movement.

But here's the truth that still hurts: for all the knowledge I've gained over the last 20 years, I couldn't find the right words to save my father. Telling someone what they should do, even when you know in your heart it would help them, can turn people off. Words are clumsy.

And I proved that.

I spent decades learning about health, fitness, and healing, yet I couldn't reach my dad in time — not before his diagnosis, not in a way that truly landed. He often told us: "God will always use you if you're usable."

He'd remind us to trust God's will, even when it makes little sense. "What father doesn't want the best for his kids?" he'd ask. "So why wouldn't the All-Father want that for us?"

I miss my dad every single day. That ache doesn't go away. But this book is my second chance. I'm writing this so you can help your dad. Possibly your mom. Wife. Husband. Kids. Neighbor. Friend. Even yourself.

I'm speaking on these pages the way I wish I could have spoken to my own father, back when it mattered most.

To my wife: Some people say they have the best spouse in the world; I know I do. My wife, Toni, is my muse.

My wife is the reason anything creative flows out of me at all. She's given me tough love when I didn't want to hear it and lifted my head when I couldn't lift it myself. She gave me three beautiful children and became the stepmother most people only dream of: fierce, loving, and ready to go to war for our family.

She is the glue that holds us together. The heart and soul of our home. She's my queen. Partner. My reason. Thank you, my love, for standing by me, even when I've been off-the-wall, extra, and hard to deal with.

To my children. Jade, Jermaine Jr., Jessi, and J'wa, who inspires me to do more.

Thank you for reminding me who I am, and whose I am. I love you.

Prologue

Not to preach. Not to claim I know it all. But to offer something that makes you pause long enough to ask, "Could this help me?" That pause, that moment of curiosity, is the seed. And once it's planted, it's only a matter of time before it grows into something that changes your life.

Let's say I break down a plant like Moringa. I talk about how it's packed with nutrients, how cultures worldwide have used it to support energy, inflammation, immune health, and more. And let's say I present it in a way that makes you stop scrolling or stop flipping pages and go, "Hold up... is that true?"

I suggest doing your own research. Investigate the studies. Read the stories. You check the sources. You learn something new, and the next thing you know, you're out in your yard planting a Moringa tree or ordering the powder to add it to your smoothies.

That's a win. That's the goal. Because when you look into things for yourself, you take your power back.

That's what this book is about. Helping you think differently. Helping you question the version of health, food, and fitness you are at, and showing you that there's a better way.

I will teach you a way that doesn't rely on broken systems, bad advice, or depending on people who don't care about your actual well-being.

I started the GrowFitFL YouTube channel to share what I've learned over the last twenty-plus years. From herbs to food forests, workouts to mental health, I've made it my mission to pass this knowledge on in a way that's real, and easy to apply, especially for families like mine raising kids, juggling bills, and trying to build something meaningful in the middle of modern chaos.

This book is not about being perfect. It's not about being extreme. It's about being intentional. Being intentional with your food. Intentional with your movements. Intentional with your environment and how you take care of your body, your mind, your home, and your people.

I'm not a doctor or a guru. I'm a man who's been through enough life to know that if you want to be self-sufficient, you better stop waiting for someone to come save you.

That's why I wrote this. Because I believe God gave us what we need. The food is in the ground. The medicine is in the leaves. Strength is in the struggle. And the future is in our hands.

This is your blueprint. Page by page. Seed by seed. Set by set. Let's grow something real.

This book is for the person who just needs that last spark to get started. It's for the one who keeps preaching to family and friends about health, fitness, and gardening but feels like nobody's listening. Sometimes the message hits differently when it comes from someone else, and I'm here to be that messenger. It's also for the person who never realized how far things have slipped until now. With the right knowledge in your hands, you can take control and start building the life you deserve.

As for how to use it: I designed this book to be practical, and easy to pick up whenever you need it. Each chapter stands on its own and gives you enough actionable information to put into practice right away. If you read just one chapter a day, you'll see a real return on that time, every single time.

Praise God,

Jermaine

GrowFitFL

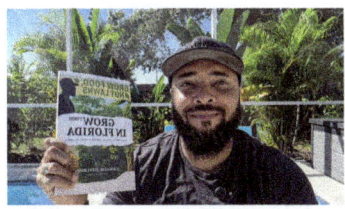

Author: Jermaine Jefferson

Introduction

This book sits at the center of everything I do with GrowFitFL. It holds the lessons that took me years to learn, the ones that only come from getting it wrong, fixing it, and doing it again. I share a lot through videos, but this book is different. This is the complete picture. No shortcuts. No theory. Just what works.

I updated this edition because of a few major storms we have had that have hurt a lot of backyard growers. Gardens change. Weather changes. People change. What worked five years ago is not always enough today. The additions in this version come from actual situations, not trends or opinions.

As I write this, Central Florida is going through one of the coldest winters we have seen in decades. Multiple nights below 30 degrees. More cold is on the way. This kind of weather is brutal on tropical fruit trees. It does not care how much money you spent or how long you waited for a harvest. Failure to prepare results in plant loss.

My wife and I have spent years figuring out how to protect what we grow. We have tested methods, failed more than once, and adjusted until we found what actually works. I included those strategies here so that the next hard winter does not surprise you. The goal is simple. Keep your trees safe. Protect your time. Protect your investment.

A lot has changed since I first wrote *Grow Food Not Lawns*. GrowFitFL has grown into one of the largest garden and health-focused YouTube channels in Central Florida. That did not happen by accident. It came from showing up daily, answering questions, and doing the work even when it was exhausting.

Between raising a family, working, caring for over 120 fruit trees, maintaining two Blue Zone-style gardens, and creating content worth watching, the days are full. I keep doing it because helping someone turn an empty yard into a source of food, health, and confidence never gets old.

Growing food changes how you live. It changes how you eat. It changes how you spend your money.

For our family of six, growing food has cut our grocery bill nearly in half. That margin matters. It means more freedom. More trips. More time with family. Less dependence on overpriced food that offers less every year.

This book is a blueprint for building that kind of life.

Inside these pages is nearly 20 years of experience. What I added in this edition doesn't replace or cancel out the first one. The original helped introduce thousands of people to gardening. This edition simply builds on that foundation, adding a few more lessons I've learned to help everyone grow stronger, more reliable gardens year-round.

Thank you for trusting me with your time. I hope this book earns its place on your shelf.

Jermaine Jefferson

Chapter 1

NOT BUILT FOR US

Let's stop calling it a broken system. It functions precisely as its creators intended, ensuring people remain tired, distracted, unhealthy, and dependent.

The year was 2020, and the world tilted. Streets went quiet. Schools and gyms closed. Governors read nightly orders on TV. By late spring, stay-at-home mandates had covered most of the country, reaching roughly seventy-three percent of U.S. counties.

California was the first state to shut down on March 19, and dozens followed through May. The message was simple: Stay inside. Figure it out. I walked into the grocery store and it felt like a movie set after the crew had left. Produce racks, stripped. Egg cases, bare.

The things that keep a family strong were gone. Managers taped paper signs to the shelves, setting limits on what you could buy. Milk, eggs, diapers, even soap. It was rationing by another name. Big retailers publicly confirmed those purchase caps as demand spiked and shelves emptied again later that year.

We all remember the signs: two per customer. Come back tomorrow. Then came the meat shock.

Processing plants went dark as workers got sick, and the numbers behind those closures were brutal. Analysts estimated capacity losses up to twenty-five percent in beef, forty-three percent in pork, and fifteen percent in chicken.

That's not a hiccup. That's a supply chain on its knees. People called it panic-buying. Psychologists called it something else: a predictable reaction to fear, scarcity, and uncertainty.

When our brain's sense threat, we try to grab control in any way we can. In 2020, that looked like carts full of paper towels and shelves of toilet paper disappearing in hours.

Studies later mapped the behavior, and the headlines turned into data. The pictures of empty aisles were not your imagination. Inside all that chaos, a different storyline started growing. Seeds. Buried under the noise was a quiet revolt that began in the backyard.

A century-old seed company, Burpee, reported the biggest spring in its history as orders exploded in March 2020.

Seed demand stayed elevated through 2021. That was a signal. Families decided they would no longer wait for the system to feed them. They were going to plant. That's when I found the phrase that reset my life: food forest. I was on YouTube, watching people stroll through their yards as if they were walking a personal market.

Mangoes in the morning. Greens in the afternoon. Herbs for tea at night. While the world argued over supply chains, these folks were harvesting dinner. The pandemic didn't control their nutrition. They even had enough to share with family and neighbors.

I stared at the screen and said it out loud: This is the way.

The feeling in my gut wasn't trendy. It was a responsibility. I'm the leader in my home. In that moment, I had no plan. That's a hard sentence to admit. I couldn't live with it. I promised my family two words: Never again. From there, it moved fast.

My wife and I started sketching a new life on notebook paper. We mapped the sun in our soon-to-be backyard. Counted water access points. Listed what our kids actually eat, not what a magazine says is cute in a raised bed.

We identified perennials that return without begging for attention and incorporated seasonal annuals. We studied how to stack layers: trees over shrubs over ground covers, so the same square footage could feed us many times a year. A garden that looks like a forest, built for Florida heat, built for storms, built to produce.

A system, not a hobby. The president declared a national emergency on March 13. Orders rolled out state by state. Limits hit stores.

Even though experts said new food products were ready, problems with getting them to stores and processing them meant we saw empty shelves. That gap between policy and pantry is where families suffer. I decided our family would close that gap ourselves.

But here's the thing: I didn't want to keep this to myself. The more I researched our food system, the deeper I went, the more I realized how many families were in the same position we were. Confused. Frustrated. Exhausted from paying more and getting less.

I felt this weight on my chest, as if I had to share what I was learning. So I started a YouTube channel called GrowFitFL.

At first, it was just me with a camera in my backyard, talking about plants. Explaining what grows well in Florida. Showing people how to plant a mango tree or grow moringa from seed. Simple stuff. Proper stuff.

But the comments started rolling in. People weren't just saying, "Thanks for the tips." They were saying things like: "I didn't know I could grow this." "My kids are eating vegetables for the first time because we grew them together." "You just saved me $200 at the grocery store this month." That's when it hit me.

This wasn't just about gardening. This was about freedom. Financial freedom. Health freedom. The independence that lets you sleep better at night knowing your family can eat, no matter what's happening in the world.

The more videos I made, the more I uncovered. I saw how our food, health, and finances are all related. And let me tell you, the deeper you look, the uglier it gets. But I'll get into that in a minute.

What matters is this: I'm not here as some guru on a mountaintop. I'm here as a dad, a husband, a regular guy who got fed up with a system that doesn't care about us. I started GrowFitFL to help people take back control of their grocery bills, health, and independence.

And if you're reading this, I'm guessing you feel the same way I did when I stood in that empty grocery store aisle. You're ready to stop waiting for someone else to fix this. You're ready to build something real. Let me show you how. I'm not a doomsday prepper.

I respect people who live prepared because they see what most ignore. The truth is simple: control what you can control. Food is not optional.

If you love your people, you build a plan that feeds them when the trucks are late, when the prices jump, when a storm knocks out power, or when the headlines say "wait." We're done waiting. This book is the blueprint I wish I had in my hands that first week I saw bare shelves.

It's for the person who knows they don't need perfection; they need progress. It will show you how to turn whatever land you have into layered nutrition.

Discover how to cultivate medicinal plants in your backyard whose names you can actually pronounce. How to push a mower less and spend more time harvesting breakfast. How to build a backyard that keeps your family strong when the world gets loud. We all have a starting point. That was mine. The world tilted. I planted my feet. Now I plant trees.

And I'm handing you the map so you can do the same. The Taste of the Problem We're living in a time when the food doesn't even look or taste the same. Tomatoes feel like rubber. Strawberries look flawless but taste like water. Bananas go from green to brown without ever being sweet.

And somehow, we're paying more than ever for all of it. This isn't just inflation. This problem affects more than one store or city. It's nationwide.

We're paying more for food that delivers less. Less nutrition. Less flavor. Smaller packaging. We're buying the same brands we always have, but now the bags are lighter, the boxes are thinner, and the price tags are higher. It's called shrinkflation.

And no, I'm not talking about a sitcom punchline. I'm talking about the same products you've bought for years now costing more and giving you less. This is real. And it's hitting families in every neighborhood, not just the ones struggling financially.

Even the cheap food, the processed filler items people used to rely on when times got hard, is now marked up so high that they're barely affordable. And families are feeling it hard. I recently spoke with a family who told me they're doing what they call "one-meal weekends."

That means on Saturdays and Sundays, they skip breakfast and lunch. The entire family of four eats only dinner. Fasting? Yes, it's healthy. I do it myself by choice. This family? Not by choice. Out of necessity.

Thankfully, their kids are in high school. Can you imagine doing that with toddlers? Imagine looking your five-year-old in the eyes and saying, "There's no breakfast today, baby. It's the weekend." That's not normal. But that's the reality some families are in right now. And I know there are families all over the world living this lifestyle daily. It sucks. And it's not just families who are barely scraping by.

One of my neighbors stopped me the other day and said, "Jermaine, I gotta talk to you." He knows what I do, and he wanted to share what his brother's going through. He said his brother and his wife both made good money. Two strong incomes. Significant cutbacks have become necessary for them recently.

They stopped eating out. I assumed it was a healthy decision. I smiled and said, "That's great, probably saving money and eating cleaner too." He shook his head. "No," he said. "They stopped eating out because they can't afford it anymore. Their grocery bill alone went up over seven hundred dollars a month. Their supplements went up another hundred. Subscriptions and gym memberships? Another three hundred fifty a month."

He said after crunching the numbers, his brother realized they were spending nearly twenty-five hundred dollars more per month than they were just a year ago. No raise. No promotion. Just higher costs everywhere. And if things don't change, they'll be in debt within fourteen months.

Then my neighbor paused and said something that hit even harder. "I did my math, man. I'm spending about nine hundred dollars more each month than I was last year. And I didn't even notice it right away. Groceries. Gas. Streaming. Electricity. Everything is up."

Then he looked me in the eye and said, "I want to start a food forest in my backyard. You were right. Prices aren't going back down. This is the new normal. I need to take some control back." That's the moment everything clicked for him.

The lightbulb moment. I've been telling the GrowFitFL community for a while now on my YouTube channel, @GrowFitFL, that this isn't temporary. This is a new baseline. And when you finally come to grips with that, you either get crushed by it... or you take your freedom back.

For my family, it started with growing food. But it didn't stop there. Food and gym memberships are no longer among our ninety-nine problems. We grow most of our produce. We eat in-season crops that are nutrient dense and taste like they came straight out of the Garden of Eden. Soon we'll have a chicken or two. Or five. Who knows? But we're not waiting for the system to feed us anymore.

We built our own. And here's the part people overlook: growing food is just one piece of the freedom equation. There are two more areas every family should secure, no matter where you live, how much space you have, or how much money you make. The first is a personal library. The second is a home gym. Build Your Library. Let's talk about the library first.

You don't need a giant room or a fancy bookshelf. A few square feet and a small stack of powerful books are enough. Create a space where knowledge lives. Books that inspire you. Books that challenge you. You can find books that will improve your mind and enrich your soul. It's one of the most underrated investments you can make.

Think about it. You have access to the thoughts, strategies, and stories of men and women who have already done what you're trying to do.

They've written how they did it so you can learn it in less time. It possesses tremendous worth. That's like mentorship, but in a book. That's wisdom on demand. Reading gives you something scrolling never will: clarity. Focus. Depth.

And right next to that library, you need a home gym. Build Your Gym. Again, I'm not talking about a garage full of expensive machines. I'm talking about making space in your home, even if it's just a corner of the living room or a section of the porch, where your body knows it's time to move. A pull-up bar. Resistance bands. A couple of dumbbells. A yoga mat. That's enough.

We now have more research proving the benefits of strength training than we have on almost any single plant you can grow in a garden. Seriously. Exercise isn't a luxury anymore. It's a necessity. Regular movement boosts your immune system, supports mental health, increases energy, reduces inflammation, builds stronger bones and muscles, and helps you stay independent as you age. It's not hype. It's science.

And when your gym is in your house, the excuses vanish. Instead of driving across town or being stuck in traffic, you'll be training at home. You're not sharing equipment with 20 other people. You're doing what you need to do in your own space, on your own time.

Your home should be your foundation.

A place to grow food.

A place to train your body.

A place to feed your mind.

That's why I say the system designers never intended for us to thrive. Because if it were, we wouldn't have to fight this hard just to afford groceries, stay healthy, and raise strong families.

But the beauty in that truth is this: once you see it, you don't have to stay stuck in it. Growing your own food is possible. Your own home is a place where you can train. You can read your own books. You can teach your kids what the world won't.

Walk into any bookstore and you will see shelves full of titles promising to motivate you, fix your habits, or change your life. There are endless books on self-help and personal development, but try finding one that teaches you how to take back control of your food.

Try finding one that shows you how to grow your own medicine right in the backyard. You won't find it. That gap has always struck me. Our ancestors did this for thousands of years, planting, harvesting, and healing with what grew around them.

Yet in our modern, developed world, we treat gardening like a hobby instead of survival.

If God grants me the clarity, this book will be the missing guide. A book to help more people return to the roots of real self-reliance. Not theory and not hype, just the practical steps to grow food and medicine the way humans have always done.

Let's jump in.

Chapter 2

THE HIDDEN COST

The Hidden Cost Have you ever eaten the same can of soup on three different days and thought, "Why does this taste different every time?" It's not in your head. Shippers often store canned food in the U.S. for weeks, months, or even years in shipping containers before it reaches consumers.

One can be relatively fresh. Another might've sat through two summers in a metal box on a dock in 100-degree heat. Same brand, same label, a completely unique experience. And that's just one example.

Food today doesn't taste the same, and more people are waking up to that truth. Strawberries look better than ever, but they're bland. Tomatoes feel like rubber. Bananas go from green to brown overnight without ever getting sweet. The flavor is fading. The nutrients are fading. But the prices? Going nowhere but up.

This isn't just inflation. It's a system problem. We're paying more for food that delivers less. We're paying more for food that is worse for us. Less nutrition. Worse flavor. Smaller portions that spent nearly half their lives in a truck, a plane, or a warehouse before landing on your plate.

That's the reality most Americans face, and it's collapsing at the seams. I did the research for a video on my channel, and what I found was shocking.

The average American meal travels about fifteen hundred miles before it ever hits your fork. Processed food averages around thirteen hundred miles. Fresh produce is closer to fifteen hundred. Fifteen hundred miles.

Think about that. Your apple takes a cross-country road trip before you bite into it. Your tomato has racked up more travel points than you did last year. And by the time it reaches you, much of the nutritional value has already faded.

Nutritionally, those miles matter. Vitamins break down the longer food sits in storage and on trucks. What should be fuel for your body becomes filler. Environmentally, it's worse. All those miles burn fuel, clog distribution centers, and pump emissions into the air. The energy it takes just to transport food is staggering, and most people never think about it.

Practically, it means every time the system hiccups, whether it's a pandemic, a storm, or a spike in fuel prices, grocery shelves go empty almost overnight. That's the world your average meal lives in.

Now imagine the alternative. That's what I show on my channel. How much control we lose when we depend on this broken system, and how quickly we can take that control back by growing even a small portion of our own food. We stop paying more for less by planting something proper right under our feet.

Shrinkflation is an actual phenomenon. They call it "shrinkflation." Same product. Smaller quantity. Higher price. One day you realize your bag of chips feels lighter. Your peanut butter jar is shorter. Your juice bottle is thinner. But the price tag went up.

This isn't a conspiracy. It's happening in plain sight, and grocery store shelves across the country are full of examples. Now add in the food miles. According to the University of Michigan, the average produce item in the

U.S. travels over 1,500 miles before it gets to you. That's gas, labor, time, packaging, and preservation costs built into your grocery bill, all of it passed down to you, the consumer.

The Dangerous Illusion of "Fresh" Even "fresh" food isn't so fresh anymore. Harvesting of the apples, tomatoes, or carrots you buy happened weeks ago. Storekeepers then stored, waxed, or gassed them to make them look fresh on the shelf. That long shelf life doesn't preserve the nutrients; it just extends appearance.

And the longer food sits in transport or storage, the more nutrients it loses. You're paying full price for half the benefit. Produce is now riskier than meat: Let's talk about food recalls. You'd think the riskiest items would be raw meat or seafood, but you'd be wrong.

According to data from PIRG and Consumer Reports, leafy greens like romaine lettuce and bagged salads are now considered the most dangerous food items in America with E. coli, Salmonella, and Listeria outbreaks.

These types of food-borne illnesses caused over 1,300 illnesses in just 13 outbreaks last year alone. Why? Because people eat salads raw, heat cannot kill the bacteria.

That steak on your plate? You likely cooked it. That bagged salad? Straight from the bag to your mouth. Canned foods are a lottery. We're also dealing with unpredictability in canned goods.

The shipping timelines, the storage conditions, and the preservatives used all affect flavor and quality. The same can of soup can taste completely different from one week to the next. That's because it may have taken a completely unique journey before you opened it.

You could eat one can that sat for 6 months and another that sat for 2 years, both with the same expiration date. And no, there's no way for you to know. So how can we trust what we're eating? This system's quality control prioritizes profit over health, so how can we rely on it? Food is getting expensive and dangerous. And now, the cost.

Even low-income families notice that "cheap food" isn't cheap anymore. One-dollar boxed meals are now two dollars. Bread is up. Milk is up. Even the discount brands have doubled. This isn't just a bump. It's a shift. A new baseline. And it's happening while food quality is dropping and health risks are rising.

Let me be clear: this is not about fear. It's about awareness.

It's about helping you recognize the pattern so you can do something about it. What you can do about it: Grow your own. Having land isn't a requirement. Even if you're in an apartment. Even if all you've got is a small balcony, a patio, or a sunny windowsill, grow something.

Begin with herbs. In cooperate some greens. Start with one pot, one plant, and one tray of microgreens. Start small, but start.

Because once you do, everything changes. You are no longer dependent on a supply chain that disregards you and no longer putting blind trust in shipping labels and packaging dates. You're no longer trading your health for convenience.

When you grow your own food, you know what went into it. The soil, water, care, and timing are all under your control. You know it hasn't been sitting on a truck for 1,500 miles. You know no one has gassed, waxed, sprayed, or irradiated it to fake its freshness.

And here's the truth: Everything you grow at home is fresher, cleaner, and more nutrient-dense than what's sitting in your store's organic section.

When you take back your food, you take back your power. And this system? Your success relies on you never doing that. It's not built for you to be self-sufficient. It's built for you to be a customer. For life. Dependent. Complacent. We are always buying and consuming, but never truly thriving. That's why growing even one tomato plant is an act of rebellion.

That's why planting herbs on your windowsill is bigger than it looks.

That's why showing your kids how to grow food isn't just cute; it's revolutionary. Because the more you grow, the less you need from them. This isn't just about saving money on groceries. This is about reclaiming your freedom, your health, and your peace of mind.

You don't need acres. You don't need to be perfect. But you need to begin. And listen closely, because this matters. The same inflation that is draining your grocery bill is now creeping into the gardening world. Fruit trees, raised beds, pots, irrigation systems — all of it is rising in price while giving you less.

Here's what I mean. Just a few years ago, you could buy a fifteen-gallon mango tree for the same price you now pay for a five-gallon tree. Same tree, same species, but smaller size at the same cost. Many nurseries are playing the same game the food system has been playing for years. Shrink the product, raise the price, and hope nobody notices.

I remember the first raised bed we bought for our garden. We loved it and wanted to match it with another a few years later. Same brand, same model, same store. But the price had doubled. Not an upgrade. Not a premium option. Just the same box at twice the cost.

I'm not saying this to state the obvious. Because what feels obvious to you and me may not be obvious to someone just getting started. The truth is simple: building your food forest today costs far more than it did when my wife and I started in 2021. And it will cost even more next year.

So now is the time. Buy your trees, your seeds, your soil, and your tools. Every month you wait, prices climb higher. Waiting only makes the hill steeper. Starting now locks in value for the future. It starts with a seed. And from that seed, you grow more than food. You develop control. Confidence is something you develop. You grow independence. You grow a legacy.

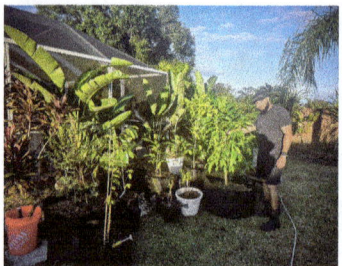

Jermaine walking through his Florida backyard food forest, showing established fruit trees and edible plants growing in real Florida conditions.

Chapter 3

YOUR HEALTH IS A GARDEN

> "And the Lord God took the man and put him into the garden of Eden to dress it and to keep it."
> –Genesis 2:15 (KJV)

From the very beginning, God didn't place man in a palace, a temple, or a battlefield. He placed him in a garden.

That tells you everything you need to know.

The garden is where we lived, moved, and thrived. This is the place where health began. It had the provision built into it. It's where work had meaning and where rest had rhythm. The garden wasn't just a location. It was a system. A blueprint for how human beings existed.

But today?

Most people are so far removed from the soil, they don't even recognize the seeds of sickness being planted in their own homes, diets, and minds. They treat their bodies like landfills, then wonder why they feel like a dump.

See, your body is a garden.

What you feed it is your seed. What do you believe? That's your sun or shade. And your habits either water your well-being or slowly dry you out.

> "Be not deceived; God is not mocked: for whatsoever a man soweth, that shall he also reap." – Galatians 6:7 (KJV)

That's not just spiritual law. It's biological.

If you sow stress, junk food, and neglect, you reap exhaustion, disease, and imbalance. But if you sow clean food, rest, movement, and peace, you give the body what it needs to remember how to heal.

Here's the problem, though: most people don't think they need a garden until they're sick.

Until they're sitting in a doctor's office asking for options.

Until they're scared.

Until they feel that first major sickness... or watch someone they love fade right in front of them.

That's the wake-up call. And I get it. I've had mine too.

But I ask: Why wait?

Why not explore what can help you before you become desperate? Why wait until your body is screaming before you decide to listen?

Imagine if we hadn't waited.

Imagine using preventative herbs and plants to build a body that can fight. A mind that can stay clear. A nervous system that knows how to calm itself. Imagine having 10, 20, 30 more healthy years with your family because you built now, not begged later.

When you're young, you feel untouchable. It feels as though you have a body made of steel, and time is on your side. You power through exhaustion and ignore the warning signs. You tell yourself you'll get to it later.

But all it takes is one scare, one ER visit, one phone call about someone you love, and everything shifts.

Suddenly, health isn't something you take for granted anymore. It becomes precious. Urgent. Personal.

So again, I ask: Why wait for your wake-up call?

It's time to build gardens. We should plant now. Let's learn now. Let's prepare while we still have breath in our lungs and energy in our bodies.

The Wake-up Call I'll Never Forget

I saw this up close after I lost my father.

That grief hit hard. It was quiet, but heavy. The kind that doesn't make a sound but changes you from the inside out. There were moments I could've slipped into numbness, moments where I didn't want to feel anything at all. But the garden wouldn't let me.

I'd go outside just to breathe. Pull a few weeds. Water something small. The sun would hit my back, and for a minute, I'd feel like I could keep going.

The garden gave me a place to grieve and grow at the same time.

It didn't fix the pain. It didn't bring him back. But it held space for me. It gave me somewhere to put my hands when my heart didn't know what to do. And somewhere in the middle of that pain, I started noticing what was growing, not just in the yard, but in my spirit.

I became more curious. More intentional. More present.

That's when I started looking deeper into medicinal plants. Not just the surface stuff. I'm talking about serious healing. Plants like moringa, anamu, ashwagandha, lemongrass, katuk, elderberry, and ginger. They didn't just help me physically. They redefined what I believed about health.

I was studying ashwagandha, researching its effects on stress, grief, cortisol, trauma, and nervous system repair. And then, knowing nothing I was working on, my wife came home with a packet of ashwagandha seeds.

I stopped.

I looked at her. She did not know why I was studying it. She just felt led to bring it home.

That wasn't a coincidence. That was God.

God always provides. Praise God.

That one act led me deeper. Diving into study. Into stewardship. Into healing. I started researching not just how to grow these plants, but why they work. They nourish the nervous system. How they help the body remember its original settings. How this knowledge has been with our ancestors all along, passed down, ignored, dismissed, and now it's making its way back to us.

> "He causeth the grass to grow for the cattle, and herb for the service of man: that he may bring forth food out of the earth." –Psalm 104:14 (KJV)

Herbs aren't extras. They're medicine.

And when you grow them yourself, when you put your own hands in the dirt, the healing hits differently. It multiplies.

Think of your gut as soil. Your thoughts are like the weather. Your rest is sunlight. Stress is the pest. Trauma is the drought.

And the answer has always been the same. The seed.

You don't need perfection to start

Here's what I want you to hear: You don't need the perfect yard. You don't need to know everything before you start. What you need is faith to plant the first one. Willingness to learn as you go.

And when you mess up, and you will, that's not failure. That's compost. That's fuel for what comes next.

Every gardener kills plants. Every single one. I've killed more plants than I can count. Over-watering can cause some issues. Some from under-watering. Some I planted in the wrong spot, at the wrong time, with the wrong expectations.

But I kept going. And you know what? The wins started outweighing the losses.

My moringa tree that survived provided shade for the backyard. The lemongrass that took off became tea for the whole family. The ginger that thrived became medicine in the cabinet and flavor in the kitchen.

You don't need a green thumb. You need a willing heart.

Because here's the part most people miss: everything essential is already free.

God made almost everything we need, and it grows if we allow it. We just forgot. We handed that knowledge over and let big business convince us it was easier to let them take care of us.

Convenience replaced wisdom.

Instead of a tree in the yard, there's a box of produce. A pill bottle instead of a plant in the garden. A drive-thru meal instead of a harvest from the backyard.

And now we're paying the price. Literally and physically.

The Ancient Wisdom We Forgot

> "Let food be thy medicine and medicine be thy food." –Hippocrates

This is one of the oldest truths in health. Hippocrates said it over two thousand years ago, but walk into any pharmacy today and you'll see proof that we forgot it.

Instead of food that heals, we're sold food that breaks us down, and then medicine to patch us back together. The idea was never supposed to be separate. What we eat should be the first line of defense for our health.

Think about it. When did we treat food and medicine as two different things?

Your great-grandmother didn't run to the pharmacy for every cough, every ache, every moment of fatigue. She had remedies in the kitchen. Ginger for nausea. Honey for a sore throat. Garlic for immunity. She knew that what you ate either built you up or tore you down.

Somewhere along the way, we lost that.

Our health is now being outsourced to individuals whose profits depend on us remaining unwell. We stopped trusting our instincts and started trusting labels. We stopped growing our food and started buying whatever was cheap and convenient.

And the results speak for themselves.

Chronic diseases are at an all-time high. Diabetes, heart disease, inflammation, autoimmune disorders. These aren't mysterious conditions that just people have. They're the result of decades of poor input. Bad food. High stress. Sedentary lifestyles. Chemical exposure.

But here's the good news: if bad inputs create bad outcomes, good inputs create excellent outcomes.

Your body wants to heal. It's designed to heal. You just have to give it what it needs.

> "The doctor of the future will give no medicine but will interest his patients in the care of the human frame, diet, and the cause and prevention of disease." – Thomas Edison

Edison said this in the early 1900s, and here we are, still waiting for that future.

But you know what? No more waiting is necessary. We can be that future. We can be the ones who choose prevention over prescriptions. Who chooses soil over supplements? Who chooses actual food over fake convenience?

Modern science proves what Edison predicted. Diet is the foundation. What we eat directly ties into chronic illnesses like diabetes, heart disease, and inflammation. The medicine is on the plate, or it's not there at all.

These words are not just philosophy. They are reality.

When you grow food that is alive and rich in nutrients, you're giving your body what no factory can replicate. Therefore, the message is more relevant than ever. Rising food prices, stripped nutrition, and chemical additives make this ancient wisdom urgent today.

Growing even a handful of herbs or trees in your backyard is not just gardening. It is healthcare.

The Voices That Changed How I See Health

When I think about voices that shook up the way we look at food and health, Dr. Sebi is one that stands out.

His uncomfortable challenges to the mainstream started a crucial discussion. He spoke about food not as calories, but as energy. He taught that when you eat living, natural foods, the body knows what to do.

Healing is straightforward. We eliminate what harms us and return to our original state.

Dr. Sebi brought into this space an unapologetic belief that disease is not random. He connected it to mucus, to the breakdown of cells, to what we put into our bodies every single day. He offered an alternative path, rooted in herbs, plants, and what grows naturally in creation.

Whether people agreed with every detail, he made healthy people again. He made us look at the plate and ask: is this giving me life, or is it taking it away?

For me, his influence was real.

He pushed me to question the system I grew up trusting. He motivated me to question why so many people are sick, why medicine is endless but cures are rare, and why the foods sold to us have had their power stripped.

His teachings planted a seed in my thinking, one that grew into how I see my garden today. Every tree, every herb, every fruit I plant is not just food. This is medicine. It's prevention. It's strength for my family.

Dr. Sebi taught me that health is not about waiting for someone else to fix you. It's about reclaiming what God already gave us.

That perspective has shaped my choices and is part of why I do what I do now.

But Dr. Sebi wasn't the only influence that reshaped my understanding of health. There was another source of wisdom that came not from books or videos, but from family.

Learning from the Culture That Never Forgot

Since being introduced to my wife's culture and her side of the family from Haiti, my understanding of herbs and healing grew even deeper.

I saw firsthand how knowledge of plants and food never left them. They didn't need to study books or look up research to justify why herbs mattered or why growing your own food was important. It was already in their hands, in their kitchens, in their backyards.

They always kept the practice.

Just like their parents and grandparents before them, they used herbs. They grew food not as a hobby but as a way of life. They knew which leaves helped with a fever. Which roots calmed the stomach? Which teas brought down inflammation?

This diet was long-term, not short-term. Survival was the key here. This was heritage.

Watching that opened my eyes even more. It reminded me that this wisdom has always been here. Some of us just have to reclaim it.

I remember the first time I watched my wife's aunt make a remedy from scratch. No measuring cups. No internet search. Just muscle memory and confidence. She moved through the process as if it were second nature, because it was.

And I realized something powerful in that moment: this is what we lost when we traded gardens for grocery stores. We didn't just lose access to fresh food. We lost the knowledge that came with it. The awareness, the confidence, and the relationship.

But here's the beautiful part: it's not gone. It's still here. It's still being practiced. And people can still learn it.

That's what I carry forward now. A mix of what I've learned through my searching, what voices like Dr. Sebi challenged me to see, and what my family from Haiti has lived out without ever needing a textbook.

It's heritage. It's survival. And it's health.

What You Can Start Today

So where do you begin?

Modestly is how you begin. You start simple. You start with one plant.

Perhaps it's basil on your windowsill. Maybe it's a moringa tree in your backyard. Maybe it's a pot of lemongrass on your patio. It doesn't matter where you start. What matters is that you start.

Because every plant you grow is a step toward independence. Every herb you harvest is a step toward healing. Every seed you plant is a declaration: I'm not waiting anymore. I'm taking my health into my own hands.

And listen, you don't have to have all the answers. It's not a requirement to know the Latin names, the perfect soil pH, or the exact watering schedule. Learn as you go. Make mistakes and adjust. You grow, literally and figuratively.

The garden is the greatest teacher I've ever had. Because plants don't grow on my timeline, it has taught me patience. It's taught me humility, because I've killed more than I've grown in the beginning. It's taught me faith, because I put a seed in the ground and trust that something will come up.

And it's taught me that health is not a destination. It's a practice. A daily choice. A long-term investment.

Supplements cannot fix an unhealthy diet. You can't out-exercise chronic stress. You can't out-medicate a toxic environment.

But you can grow your way back to health. At a time, one plant. One meal at a time. One choice at a time.

Your Body Is Waiting

Your body is not your enemy. It's not broken beyond repair. It's not too late.

Your body resembles a garden, and you can always restore gardens.

Despite years of feeding it junk, even if you've ignored the warning signs. Even if you've been told there's no hope, your body still wants to heal. It's designed to heal. You just have to give it what it needs.

Clean water. Actual food. Sunlight. Movement. Rest. Connection.

These aren't luxuries. They're requirements.

And the good news is, you don't need a prescription for any of them. You don't need insurance approval. You don't need permission.

You just need to begin.

Plant the seed. Water the soil. Trust the process.

And watch what grows.

Because I promise you this: when you treat your body like the garden it is, everything changes.

Your energy transforms, mind becomes clear, your stress goes down, your strength increases, and your family notices. Your future opens up.

And you realize that the power to heal was never in someone else's hands. It was always in yours.

So let's build gardens now. Let's plant now. Let's learn now.

Let's grow our way back to health.

Together.

Chapter 4

NOBODY'S COMING TO SAVE YOU

Nobody's coming to save you.

Let's start there.

Prayer can be a source of help for you. It's okay to wish for things to be easier. It's possible to hope that someone arrives with the answers. But at some point, look around and realize it's on you.

What you eat, how you live, what you're building, that's all you.

And I know that's a hard truth to swallow. Society has conditioned us to wait. We should wait for the doctor to fix us. Wait for the government to protect us. Wait for the perfect moment when everything finally lines up.

But at that moment? It's not coming.

The system's purpose is not to save you. It's designed to keep you dependent. To keep you sick enough to need their solutions, but well enough to keep working, keep buying, keep consuming.

So if you're waiting for rescue, you're going to be waiting a long time.

The Wake-Up Call Most People Ignore

People wait too long to take their lives seriously.

They waited for the diagnosis. The breakdown. The warning from the doctor that makes their stomach drop. Then it's panic mode. Scrambling for answers. Googling symptoms at 2 a.m. Calling everyone they know for advice.

But by then, damage had already been done.

I'm trying to get you to see it before that moment comes. Prior to the scare. Before the emergency. Before you're sitting in a hospital room wishing you'd done things differently.

Because here's the truth: your body has been giving you signals for years.

The tiredness you blamed on being busy. That stubborn weight you couldn't seem to lose. The mental cloudiness, aches, mood swings, gut issues, constant colds.

Those weren't just random inconveniences. That was your body trying to tell you something.

And most people ignore it until they can't anymore.

I don't want that to be you.

Taking control doesn't mean doing everything all at once. It means doing something. A single decision. One habit. One step.

That's where it starts.

People build control; they don't find it. This is about training. Repetition is what it is. It's showing up even when you don't feel like it. It's not about perfection; it's about showing up even when life hits hard.

That's how you build roots.

The Contradiction Most People Live

People say they want peace, but live in chaos.

Despite saying they want to feel better, they refuse to make any changes. Although they look at wellness content, they continue to eat junk food.

They bought the gym membership but never go. They complain about being tired but stay up scrolling until midnight.

And I get it. Change is hard. Habits are sticky. Life is overwhelming.

But at some point, ask yourself: what's harder? Making the change now, or living with the consequences later?

You won't succeed if you're unwilling to do the hard work.

And you can't keep blaming the system while you're still buying into it every day. You can't curse the food industry while you're still eating their processed garbage. You can't complain about healthcare costs while you're ignoring the free medicine growing in the dirt.

That's the hard truth nobody wants to hear.

But I'm not here to make you comfortable. I'm here to wake you up.

A Message for Those Who Think Money Is the Answer

Now let me talk to the folks who've done well financially.

Maybe you've got money where food prices don't shake you. The cushion belongs to you. You've got options. You can afford organic, grass-fed, free-range, whatever label makes you feel safe.

But don't think this message isn't for you.

It is.

Because money won't save your body. Money cannot shield you from disease. You can't outsource your discipline. You can't write a check to fix what years of neglect have done to your health.

I remember hearing a preacher once say, "If money or a man can solve your problem, then you don't really have a problem."

That hit me hard.

Because the actual problems, the ones that actually matter, are deeper than your bank account.

Health. Energy. Clarity. Peace. Your body failing with no warning. While you're still booking vacations and writing checks, your immune system is failing. Your kids watching you struggle through what should be your prime years.

Money can't fix that.

I've met people with all the resources in the world but no clue what's in their food. They think just because it says organic, it's clean. Because it came in fancy packaging, it's safe. Because they paid top dollar, it's worth it.

You trust that? I don't. Not after everything we've seen.

Companies are lying. Labels are twisted. Farmers are doing things more cheaply to meet the demand. Companies buy and sell certifications. And people are still just buying and hoping.

Hoping that someone else did their job right. Hoping that the system they already know, which is broken, worked correctly this time.

That's not a strategy. That's a gamble.

That's why I say this is bigger than the budget. It's about control. Proper control.

Knowing what's in your soil. What's on your food? What you're feeding your family. That starts with growing something yourself.

Why Fresh Matters More Than You Think

And don't get it twisted. Even the so-called "good stuff" loses power when it's been sitting around.

Herbs lose strength when they're sitting in a warehouse for weeks. Picked. Dried. Packed. Shipped from who-knows-where. By the time that bag of powder hits your doorstep, it's not the same. Not even close.

A decrease in enzyme activity is being observed. The nutrients are degrading. The life force, if you want to call it that, is gone.

But when you grow the same plant in your yard? Pick it fresh? Use it fresh? You feel the difference. It works differently.

It's not a placebo effect. That's not dreaming. That's how God designed it.

Fresh food has a vitality that processed food, no matter how expensive, can never replicate. It is a living thing, and it's potent. It's working with your body, not against it.

So, to my wealthy readers, I'm telling you straight: use your money wisely.

Don't just collect things. Build something that gives back.

A home garden is one of the smartest investments you can make. Not just for food, but for healing, security, and peace of mind.

Spend the money on good soil. Quality seeds. Fruit trees that will feed your family for decades. Pay someone to help you set it up if you need to. Hire a landscaper who knows food forests, not just ornamental plants.

It's worth it.

Because what's coming down the road? The increasing expenses and supply chain disruptions. The uncertainty.

You'll want to be ready.

And a garden isn't just insurance. It's freedom. It's knowing that no matter what happens out there in the world, your family can still eat.

That's power money can't buy. But money can help you build it.

For everyone else grinding every day

And for everyone else, the rest of us, the ones grinding, working long hours, barely catching a break, this message is for you too.

Actually, it's especially for you.

Don't think just because your space is small, or your budget is tight, that this life isn't for you. Don't let anyone tell you that growing food is only for people with acres and money to burn.

I've seen people grow actual food in old buckets. Milk crates. Broken pots. Five-gallon containers from the hardware store.

I've seen folks flip a patch of dirt in the side yard into a food source that feeds them year-round.

I've seen single moms with three kids, working two jobs, still make time to plant something. Not because they had extra time. Because they made it a priority.

So miss me with the excuses.

You don't have space? Grow vertically. Use containers. Hang pots from the porch.

You don't have time? Start small. One plant. Five minutes a day.

You don't have money? Seeds are cheap. You can create soil. You can find containers.

You don't have experience? Nobody does at first. You learn by doing.

The only thing stopping you is you.

You start with what you've got. A balcony. A windowsill. An old container. Whatever.

You don't need a green thumb. You need a reason.

And if your health, your peace, your future, your family aren't reason enough, then you're not ready yet.

But I'm still going to tell you the truth, anyway.

Because one day you will be ready. And when that moment comes, I want you to remember this chapter. I want you to know that it's possible. That people with less than you have done it. That you can too.

This isn't about perfection

This isn't about perfection. It's about not being soft. Not folding when life gets loud.

It's about doing what needs to be done, even when nobody's watching. Even when you're tired. Even when it feels like it doesn't matter.

Because it matters.

The planting of every seed holds importance. Your meals are important. Every skill you learn matters. Every day you choose yourself, your health, your family over convenience, that matters.

I'm not writing this from a perfect life. I'm not some guru on a mountain with everything figured out.

I'm raising children. Working. Planting in the Florida heat. Learning as I go. Messing up. Killing plants. Trying again.

I don't have all the answers. But I have enough to know that this works.

I'm doing what I can with what I have, and I'm showing other people how to do it too.

That's why I created my YouTube channel.

It's to show real people what's possible.

If you've been reading this and you're ready to stop watching and start doing, come find me at youtube.com/GrowFitFL.

I put everything out there. The work, the mistakes, and the wins. Both the times when everything thrives. And the days when everything dies.

Because this isn't a trend for me. It's life.

And I want it for you, too.

I want you to feel what it's like to walk outside and pick your breakfast. To know exactly what's in your food. To show your kids that you don't need a store to survive.

I want you to have the peace that comes from knowing your family can eat, no matter what.

That's freedom.

That's power.

That's what we're building here.

Your mistakes are part of the process

So I'll end this section like this: If you mess up? Good.

That is compost. What that is, is fuel. That's how you learn.

Every gardener kills plants. Every single one. I've killed more than I can count. Overwatered. Under-watered. This isn't the correct location. Wrong season. Wrong expectations.

But every plant I killed taught me something. And eventually, the wins started adding up.

The moringa that survived transformed into medicine. The lemongrass that grew became tea, and the ginger that thrived became both flavor and healing.

You don't need to get it perfect. You just need to start.

And when you fail, because you will, you dust yourself off and plant another one.

Garden building is driven by that mentality. That builds health. That builds legacy.

The Garden Always Gives Back

We plant with hope, sowing each seed into soil that nurtured and fed us.

The roots run deep, drawing life from the earth, while sunshine and rain work together to help every sprout bloom.

We prune to shape. Water to sustain. Compost to enrich.

Each harvest is more than food. It's a promise kept. A reminder that when we cultivate with care, the garden will always give back abundance.

But here's what most people don't realize: the garden gives back more than food.

It gives back time. Because you're not driving to the store for herbs you can pick in 30 seconds.

It gives money back. Because that $4 bunches of basil at the grocery store? You can grow $50 worth in one pot.

It gives back health. Because fresh food from your yard has more nutrients than anything shipped across the country.

It gives back peace. Because there's something deeply grounding about putting your hands in the soil.

It gives back a purpose. Because you're not just consuming anymore. You are creating, providing, and building something real.

And it gives back legacy. Because your kids are watching. They're learning. They're seeing that their family doesn't need to depend on a broken system to survive.

That's what you're really planting. Not just seeds. But a way of life.

What Comes Next?

You've made it this far for a reason.

Something inside you knows there's more. Better health. More freedom. More connection to the earth than the world has been selling you.

From here on, every page will hand you a tool, an idea, or a seed to plant in your own life.

This isn't just about gardening. It's about reclaiming what's yours.

Food that's real. Skills that last. A legacy you can see growing right in front of you.

But here's what I need you to understand: reading this book won't change your life.

Acting on it will.

You can read each chapter. Highlight every line. Nod along with every point. But if you don't actually plant something, if you don't actually make a change, nothing will be different.

Knowledge without action is just entertainment.

And I didn't write this to entertain you. I wrote this to equip you.

So as you move forward through these pages, I want you to ask yourself one question with every chapter:

"What's the one thing I can do today because of what I just read?"

Not tomorrow. Not next week. Today.

Perhaps it is ordering seeds. Maybe it's clearing a space in your yard. Maybe it's watching one video on my channel about how to plant your first tree.

It doesn't matter what it is. What matters is that you do something.

Because that's how people build gardens. Just one action at a time. One choice at a time. One seed at a time.

And before you know it, you'll look around and realize you've built something real. This will be something for your nourishment. Something that heals you. Something that lasts.

Keep going.

The next chapters aren't just something to read. They're something to live for.

Now it's time to get to work.

Chapter 5

START WHERE YOU ARE

When I first started, I was more concerned with keeping the grass cut than growing anything useful.

The mower was my most-used tool. I spent hours sweating in the Florida sun, pushing that thing back and forth across the yard, just to make sure the neighbors didn't complain about the length of my lawn.

And let me tell you, in Florida, grass grows fast. You blink and it's back. You cut it Saturday, and by Wednesday it's already creeping up again. It never stops. It's relentless.

So there I was, week after week, pouring time and energy into something that gave me nothing back. Food is unavailable. No shade. No medicine. Just a green carpet that needed constant attention.

And yet, when I look back at that season of my life, I realize I was spending all that time and energy keeping something alive that could never feed me.

I understood the irony.

My father used to say the same thing about work. How people grind themselves down for a paycheck that never really fills them. A lawn is no different. It gives nothing back.

It just takes. The time that belongs to you. Your gas. Your weekends. And for what? So it can look like everyone else's yard?

That's when it hit me. I was working for the grass. The grass wasn't working for me.

And if I were going to sweat in this Florida heat anyway, I might as well be growing something that mattered.

The first step is always ugly

I remember the first time I broke that cycle. It wasn't dramatic. No big moment. No earth-shattering revelation.

I just planted two small trees.

Two scraggly, sad-looking things I picked up from a local nursery. I didn't know how to care for them. I watered them too much at first, then not enough. I mulched them wrong. Put them in spots that got too much sun, then move them to spots that didn't get enough.

They looked pitiful most of the time. Honestly, I thought they were going to die.

But they survived.

And that survival taught me more than the thousand times I had thought about starting and never did.

To start, I discovered that flawless technique wasn't a requirement. I didn't need to know everything. I didn't need ideal conditions or a master plan.

I just needed to look foolish and keep showing up.

Those two trees gave me the courage to plant more. Without them, nothing you see in my yard today would exist.

That means it's not the moringa. Not the papayas. Not the sweet potatoes, nor the lemongrass, nor the katuk. None of it.

It all started with two trees I almost killed.

And here's what I want you to hear: your first step doesn't have to be perfect either.

In fact, it won't be. It can't be. Because you don't know what you don't know yet.

But that's okay. That's part of it. That's how you learn.

You are planting. I will show you. You adjust. You try again.

And slowly, piece by piece, you figure it out.

The Stories That Prove It's Possible

I've met so many people over the years who thought they couldn't start because their situation wasn't ideal.

They have no land of their own. Fixed income. No time. No experience.

But let me tell you about some folks who proved all of that wrong.

There was Ruth. A woman in her seventies, living on nothing but Social Security in a little apartment in Clearwater. She didn't have land. What she had were two cracked storage bins she found behind a Dollar General.

She filled those bins with soil and set them on her porch. Grew collards, basil, and peppers in those bins.

And I'll never forget what she told me when I visited her. She said, "Jermaine, I never felt rich until I saw the leaves rising out of that soil."

She gave bags of collards to her neighbors. People who had yards twice the size of hers but never thought to grow a thing.

Ruth didn't let her situation stop her. She worked with what she had. And it was enough.

Then there was Miguel in Tampa. Renting a duplex with a patch of dirt in the back that was too sandy to hold water. He wanted a mango tree, but his landlord would never allow it in the ground.

So, you know what he did? He put one in a twenty-five-gallon pot.

For two years, he watered it. Mulched it. Moved it around the yard, chasing the sun. People laughed at him. Told him it would never work. Told him he was wasting his time.

Then, one summer afternoon, he sent me a picture. He is holding his first mango from that tree. The biggest smile I'd ever seen on his face.

He told me it was the best fruit he'd ever tasted. Not because it was sweeter or juicier than the ones from the store. But because it was his.

He was the one who grew it and nurtured it. He waited for it. And when it finally came, it was worth every drop of sweat.

That's the thing about growing your own food. It hits differently. It tastes different. Because you know the story behind it.

Starting in the Middle of Chaos

I've also seen young families with toddlers and newborns who swear they don't have time for a garden.

"Jermaine, I can barely keep up with the laundry. How am I supposed to grow food?"

I get it. Life is loud. Kids are demanding. There's always something that needs attention.

But I watched one couple plant a single papaya tree in the corner of their yard just to humor me. They didn't think it would change anything. It was just one tree.

Six months later, they were slicing papayas for breakfast while their toddler ate them straight from the peel. That tree became the spark that led them to plant guavas, lemongrass, and sweet potatoes.

They didn't wait for a season of rest. They didn't wait for the kids to get older or for life to calm down.

They started in the middle of the chaos. And life adjusted around their garden.

Because here's the truth: there's never going to be a perfect time. Life is always going to be demanding. There's always going to be something in the way.

But if you wait for the perfect moment, you'll be waiting forever.

You start now. With what you have. Within the chaos. In the chaos. In the middle of everything else.

And you figure it out as you go.

What My Kids Taught Me

Even in my home, the lesson repeats itself.

I've had my kids plant seeds in paper cups. Watching those little sprouts push through the soil, reaching for the light.

They didn't care that the seeds were uneven or the cups too shallow. They didn't worry about drainage or soil pH or any of that.

They only cared that something alive grew because of their hands.

And you should've seen their faces when those sprouts broke through. Pure joy. Pure wonder.

Those brief experiments in paper cups turned into actual gardens later. Now, when I walk through my food forest and see my children grabbing leaves of katuk or pulling carrots, I know they'll never forget what it feels like to eat food they grew.

That doesn't start with land. That starts with a paper cup and a handful of dirt.

That starts with a parent willing to let them try. To let them get dirty. To let them fail and try again.

Because you're not just teaching them how to grow food. You're teaching them how to be self-sufficient. How to not depend on a system that doesn't care about them. How to take care of themselves and the people they love.

That's a lesson worth more than any degree or credential.

Breaking Every Excuse

The point is not perfection. The point is to plant one thing.

Every excuse we make sounds reasonable until the first harvest proves it false.

Too old? Ruth proved that wrong in her seventies.

Too busy? That young couple with kids proved that wrong.

Too broke? Seeds cost a dollar. You can find soil. You can improvise pots.

Too small a space? Balconies work. Windowsills work. Storage bins work.

Too bad the soil? Amend it. Or grow in containers.

Is the landlord strict? Grow in pots. Move them if you have to.

I've heard them all, and I've watched people break them all.

The only thing that matters is putting something in the ground, or in a pot, and watching it grow.

And listen, I know Florida has its challenges. It's intensely hot. The bugs are incredibly persistent, and the sandy soil doesn't hold water. The hurricanes come through and knock everything down.

But you know what? Florida also has year-round growing. We don't have a winter that shuts everything down. We can grow food twelve months out of the year if we know what we're doing.

That's a gift most places don't have.

So yeah, we've got challenges. But we've also got opportunities. And I'd rather work with what we've got than wish I lived somewhere else.

Changing Your Relationship with Possibility

Starting where you are is not about gardening alone. It's about changing your relationship with possibilities.

It's about looking at your space, your time, your resources, and asking, "What can I do with this?"

Instead of focusing on what you don't have, you see what you have. And you make it work.

I've had neighbors laugh when I planted mango trees in sandy soil. "That'll never work, Jermaine. You're wasting your time."

Years later, those same neighbors asked for fruit.

I've had family wonder if spending weekends mulching was a waste of time. "You're out there in the heat for what? A few tomatoes?"

Now they come over for dinners made almost entirely from the yard. They see the baskets of sweet potatoes. The bunches of katuk. The bags of moringa leaves.

And they don't laugh anymore.

Each step I took, awkward and imperfect, opened doors I didn't even know were there.

Open the doors to better health. Strategies for lowering grocery costs. Doors to skills I never thought I'd have. Doors to conversations with people who wanted to learn what I was doing.

And it all started with a willingness to try. To look foolish. To plant something, I didn't know how to grow it.

Your backyard is more than decoration

That's why this chapter matters.

If you never plant that first seed, you never feel the shift. You never understand that your backyard is more than decoration. That your balcony is more than a place to store a chair. That your porch is more than a spot for the mailman.

It's potential.

If you allow it, every inch of that space can work for you. Every corner, strip of grass, and sunny spot.

This can both feed and heal you. It can teach your kids, and it can save you money. It can give you peace.

But only if you use it.

Every tree in my yard today, every basket of sweet potatoes, every papaya hanging low in the summer sun, began with an imperfect start.

I almost killed this scraggly little tree. It started as a seed I planted wrong. A pot I set in the wrong spot.

But I kept going. I kept adjusting. I kept learning.

And now, years later, I have a food forest that feeds my family. Not perfectly. Not every single meal. But enough to make a real difference.

Enough to know that if the grocery stores ran out tomorrow, we'd be okay.

Enough to teach my kids that we don't need the system to survive.

Enough to give me peace in a world that feels more uncertain every day.

The Choice You Have Right Now

So I'm asking you to stop waiting.

Stop waiting for the perfect moment. The perfect setup. The perfect knowledge.

Pick one plant. Just one.

Basil in a pot. Lemongrass by the porch. A papaya in the yard's corner. A tomato plant in a container.

Whatever you can do now, do it.

That one plant will change how you see your space. It'll change how you see yourself. It'll change what you think is possible.

And a year from now, you'll either have a story about what grew, or a story about how you waited.

Which story do you want to tell?

I know which one I'd pick. And I think you do too.

So let's do this. Let's plant something. Let's start where we are, with what we have, and see what happens.

Because I promise you, once you start, you won't want to stop.

What Comes Next?

Here's where the path leads.

Once you take that first step, once you start with what you have, the question becomes: how do you keep it alive? How do you build not just a season of food but a rhythm that feeds you every month of the year?

That's what comes next.

In the following chapter, we're going to walk together into the blueprint for a year-round garden. A food forest that works with the land instead of against it. A system that doesn't quit when summer ends or when the rain stops.

If this chapter is about planting hope, the next is about reaping security.

Start where you are today, because tomorrow we learn how to carry it through all year.

But before you turn that page, I need you to do something.

Reader's Assignment: Claim Your Space

Before you move forward, I want you to take twenty minutes and do this simple assignment.

I'm serious. Don't just keep reading. Do this.

Grab a notebook.

Then step outside and look at your space. Really look at it.

Write three things:

1. Where the sun hits in the morning, where it hits at noon, and where it fades in the evening.

This matters more than you think. Sun patterns determine what you can grow and where. You don't need to be exact. Just notice. Where does the light shine? What part does the shade cover? Where does it shift throughout the day?

2. One spot you could plant something this week.

Not someday. This week. Even if it's just a pot on a balcony or a corner of the yard. Find one spot. Claim it. That's your starting point.

3. Three foods you and your family actually eat often.

Think in meals, not plants. Pasta with basil. Smoothies with mango. Sweet potatoes roasted for dinner. Salads with tomatoes and cucumbers. Whatever you actually eat, write it down.

Then sketch a quick map of your yard or balcony.

You do not need any art skills. Just boxes and circles. Rough shapes. Arrows pointing to the sun.

Mark where you think each food could grow. That could be the spot where the basil pot sits. Where that papaya tree could go. Where those sweet potatoes could sprawl.

If you're up north, add a note about where you might place a small greenhouse, a row cover, or even a sunny window for herbs.

This is not about getting it perfect. It's about claiming the ground.

By the time you open the next chapter, you won't just be reading about a year-round garden. You'll already have your first blueprint in your hands.

That paper sketch, those three foods, and that one planting spot are the foundation. The next chapter builds the walls and the roof.

Your Garden Blueprint Starts Here

Now use this spot right here in the book to sketch your garden.

Ebook viewers, take out some paper.

Don't overthink it. Rough boxes for beds. Circles for trees. Arrows for the sun.

No one but you will see it. This isn't for show. This is for you.

What matters is that you claim the space on paper before you put it in the ground.

If you live up north, mark where you might set a small greenhouse, a row cover, or even a sunny window for herbs.

If you're in Florida like me, mark where you'll catch the most sun without frying your plants in July.

If you're in an apartment, sketch your balcony or your windowsills.

Whatever your space is, draw it. Own it. See it for what it can become.

Because once you see it on paper, once you make it real in your mind, the next step becomes obvious.

And that's when the magic starts.

That's when you stop being someone who wants to grow food and start being someone who does.

So, grab that pen. Step outside. Look at your space with fresh eyes.

And let's build something real.

Chapter 6

YEAR ROUND GARDEN

Let me be straight with you.

This chapter is the one you take notes. The one you come back to. The one you will use for years to come.

Because everything until now has been about why. You need to start, and the system is broken because... and why cultivating food is important.

This chapter is about how.

How to actually build a garden that feeds you every single month of the year. Not just summer. Not just when conditions are perfect. Every. Single. Month.

And if you're in Florida, or anywhere in zones 9-10, you're sitting on a goldmine and don't even know it.

While the rest of the country buries itself under snow, battles frost, and waits for spring, we plant. We're harvesting. We're growing food in December, January, and February.

That's power.

But only if you know how to work with Florida's rhythm instead of fighting against it.

So let's get into it. I'm going to walk you through everything. And I mean everything. By the time you finish this chapter, you'll know exactly what to plant, when to plant it, how to care for it, and how to deal with every challenge Florida throws at you.

This is the chapter you came here for. So let's make it count.

Understanding Florida's Unique Climate

First, forget everything you've learned about the four seasons. If you moved here from up north, erase that mental calendar. It doesn't apply.

In Florida, we don't have spring, summer, fall, and winter the way the rest of the country does.

We have two seasons: the wet and the dry season .

And understanding this difference is absolutely critical. Because if you try to garden here using a northern calendar, you're going to fail. You're going to plant tomatoes in July and wonder why they die. You're going to expect greens to grow in August and get frustrated when they bolt.

So let me break it down clearly.

The wet season (May to October)

This is our summer. But it's not like summer anywhere else.

The wet season's defining characteristic is afternoon thunderstorms that roll through like clockwork. Around 2 or 3 p.m., the sky darkened. The wind picked up. And then it dumps rain for 20 minutes to an hour before clearing up again.

The humidity during this time sits somewhere between oppressive and unbearable. We're talking 80-90% humidity on most days. Your shirt sticks to your back the moment you step outside.

Everything grows fast during the wet season. I mean everything. Your grass shoots up overnight. Weeds explode. Trees push fresh growth constantly.

But the heat and moisture also bring challenges. Pests multiply like crazy. Fungal diseases spread. Some plants bolt or burn out. And if your soil doesn't drain well, you'll have standing water that drowns your crops.

The wet season is not a lost cause. You can absolutely grow food during this time. But you need to pick the right plants and manage water carefully.

The dry season (November to April)

This is our "winter," but it's really our prime growing season.

The temperature drops into a comfortable range. We're talking 60s and 70s during the day, 40s and 50s at night. Some years we get a freeze or two in North Florida, but most of South Florida stays above freezing all winter.

The afternoon thunderstorm stopped. Rain becomes less frequent. The humidity backs off. And suddenly, gardening feels easy again.

The bugs slow down. Fungal diseases disappear. And your cool-season crops, tomatoes, peppers, greens, absolutely thrive.

It's the season to stock up. Most people produce your food around this time. Florida gardeners earn their money.

Understanding this rhythm changes everything.

Because in Florida, you're not trying to extend summer like northern gardeners do. You're trying to maximize the dry season and strategically manage the wet season.

Once that clicks, everything else falls into place.

The Three Layers of a Florida Food Forest

A food forest is not a traditional garden with neat rows and tilled beds. It's not a raised bed with tomatoes lined up like soldiers.

A food forest is a system that mimics how nature actually works. Multiple layers of plants growing together, feeding the soil, shading each other, supporting each other, creating a self-sustaining ecosystem.

And in Florida, this approach works better than anything else. Because once you build it right, it requires way less water, way less fertilizer, and way less work than a traditional garden.

Here are the three essential layers you need to understand.

Layer 1: The Canopy (Your Fruit Trees)

This is your long-term investment. The trees that will feed your family for decades.

These trees are the foundation of your food forest. They provide shade, fruit, and structure. They're also the slowest layer to establish, which is why you plant them first.

Even if you do nothing else, get trees in the ground. Because a tree you plant today will feed your kids five years from now. And their kids twenty years from now.

That's a legacy.

Let me walk you through the best fruit trees for Florida, zone by zone, with real details you can use.

Mango

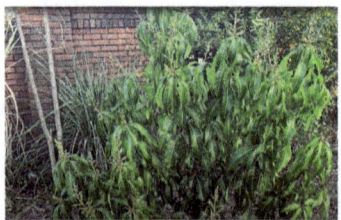

Mango Tree

Zones: 9B-10 (some varieties tolerate 9A with protection)

Mangoes are the crown jewel of Florida food forests. Once established, a single tree can produce hundreds of pounds of fruit every summer.

Planting: Full sun. Give it space, at least 25-30 feet from other trees and structures. Mangoes get big.

Soil: They prefer well-drained soil but can tolerate a range of conditions. If you've got heavy clay or standing water, plant on a mound.

Varieties to consider:

- 'Nam Doc Mai': Thai variety, sweet, fiberless, does well in South Florida
- 'Ice Cream': Classic Florida mango, super sweet, minimal fiber
- 'Carrie': Smaller tree, works in North Florida, disease-resistant
- 'Kent': Large fruit, late season, good producer

When they fruit: Late spring through summer (May-August, depending on variety)

Beginner tip: Buy a grafted tree from a reputable nursery. Don't grow from seed. A grafted tree will fruit in 2-3 years. A seed-grown tree takes 5-8 years and might not taste good.

Avocado

Zones: 9-10 (cold-hardy varieties can push into 8B)

Avocados love Florida, but they're picky about drainage. If water sits around their roots, they'll develop root rot and die.

Planting: Full sun to partial shade. Plant on a mound or raised bed if your soil holds water.

Soil: Must drain well. If you dig a hole and it fills with water during the wet season, that spot won't work for avocados.

Varieties to consider:

- 'Lula': Cold-hardy, good for North Florida
- 'Brogdon': Also cold-hardy, smaller fruit
- 'Hass' types: Work in South Florida but struggle with cold
- 'Choquette': Large fruit, great flavor, handles Florida humidity

When they fruit: Depends on the variety. Some fruit in summer, others in fall/winter.

Beginner tip: Avocados need good drainage more than they need good soil. If you've got sandy soil, perfect. If you've got clay, build a mound at least 12 inches high and 3 feet wide before planting.

Papaya

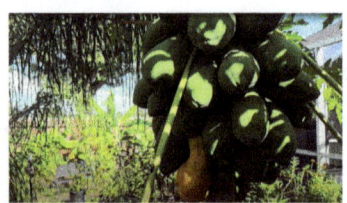

Red Lady Papaya

Zones: 9-10 (dies back in freezes but can regrow from roots in 9B)

Papayas are your quick win. You plant one today, and you're eating fruit in 9 to 12 months. No joke.

Planting: Full sun. They love heat. Space them 8 to 10 feet apart.

Soil: They tolerate poor soil as long as it drains.

Varieties to consider:

- 'Red Lady': (My Favorite) Hybrid, consistent producer, sweet fruit
- 'Maradol': Large fruit, common in Mexican markets
- 'Tainung': Productive, disease-resistant

When they fruit: Year-round in South Florida. Spring through fall in North Florida.

Beginner tip: Papayas are **male, female, or hermaphrodite (self-fertile). You want hermaphrodites because they pollinate themselves. Plant at least 2-3 to ensure you get fruit. Once they flower, you can tell which ones are which and remove the males if needed.**

Citrus

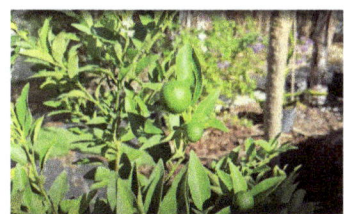

Citrus Tree

Zones: 8B-11 (depending on variety)

People know Florida for citrus. And for good reason. These trees are productive, relatively easy, and give you fruit in the winter when most other things aren't producing.

Planting: Full sun. Space 12 to 15 feet apart.

Soil: They like slightly acidic soil and good drainage.

Varieties to consider:

- Lemons ('Meyer', 'Eureka'): Year-round production

- Limes ('Key Lime', 'Persian'): Multiple harvests per year

- Oranges ('Valencia', 'Navel'): Winter harvest

- Grapefruit ('Ruby Red', 'Oro Blanco'): Winter harvest

- Tangerines ('Honey', 'Dancy'): Winter harvest

When they fruit: Most citrus fruits in winter (November-March)

Beginner tip: Citrus greening disease is a serious issue in Florida. Buy disease-free trees from certified nurseries. Don't buy citrus from random roadside stands or bring trees from other states.

Loquat

Zones: 8-10

Loquats are one of the most underrated fruit trees in Florida. They're cold-hardy, productive, and fruit in late winter to early spring when almost nothing else is producing.

Planting: Full sun to partial shade. Space 15 to 20 feet apart.

Soil: Tolerates a wide range of soil types.

Varieties to consider:

- 'Big Jim': Large fruit, sweet

- 'Oliver': self-fertile, consistent producer

When they fruit: Late winter to early spring (February-April)

Beginner tip: The fruit ripens unevenly, so you'll be harvesting over several weeks. Birds love them, so you might need to net the tree or share the harvest.

Mulberry

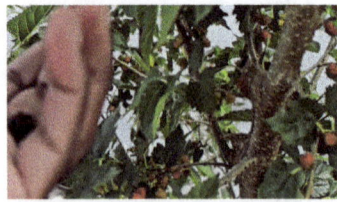

Mulberry Tree

Zones: 4-10

Mulberries are ridiculously easy. They grow fast, tolerate neglect, produce tons of fruit, and kids absolutely love them.

Planting: Full sun. Space 20-30 feet apart (they get big).

Soil: Tolerates everything, even heavy clay.

Varieties to consider:

- 'Illinois Everbearing': Large fruit, long harvest season
- 'Dwarf Everbearing': Smaller tree, good for limited space

When they fruit: Spring (March-May)

Beginner tip: Mulberries stain everything. Don't plant them over driveways, patios, or anywhere you care about purple stains. But the fruit is* delicious, *and the kids will eat* it *straight off the tree.

Banana

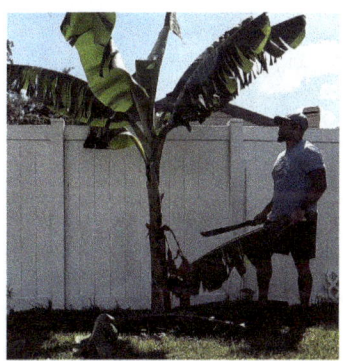

Banana Plant

Zones: 8-11 (some varieties can handle light freezes)

Bananas aren't technically trees; they're giant herbs. But they grow tall and produce tons of food, so they fit in the canopy layer.

Planting: Full sun. They love water and heat. Space 8 to 10 feet apart.

Soil: Rich, well-amended soil. They're heavy feeders.

Varieties to consider:

- 'Dwarf Cavendish': Classic banana flavor, 6-8 feet tall

- 'Ice Cream' (Blue Java): Cold-hardy, tastes like vanilla ice cream

- 'Manzano': Short, cold-hardy, sweet fruit

When they fruit: Year-round in South Florida. Spring through fall in North Florida.

Beginner tip: *After a banana plant fruits, it dies back. But it sends up fresh shoots (called pups) that become the next generation. Cut down the old stalk and let the pups grow. One plant becomes many*.

Planting Your Trees: The Step-by-Step Process

Alright, you've picked your trees. Now let's plant them right.

Step 1: Dig the hole

Make it twice as wide as the root ball, but only as deep. You want the tree sitting at the same level it was in the pot, not deeper.

In Florida's sandy soil, this is easy. In clay, it's harder. Take your time.

Step 2: Amend the soil (lightly)

Don't go crazy here. Mix some compost into the soil you removed from the hole, but don't fill the hole with pure compost. You want the roots to grow into the native soil, not stay in a compost bubble.

Step 3: Plant the tree

Remove the tree from its pot carefully. If the roots are circling, gently tease them apart. Set the tree in the hole and backfill with your amended soil.

Step 4: Water deeply

Drench the area. You want water reaching the bottom of the root ball.

Step 5: Mulch

Put down 3-4 inches of mulch around the tree, but keep it a few inches away from the trunk. Mulch touching the trunk causes rot.

Step 6: Water consistently for the first year

This is critical. The first year is all about establishing roots. Water deeply 2-3 times per week during dry periods. Once the tree establishes roots (after about a year), you can back off.

<u>Common mistake: People plant the tree too deeply. If you bury the trunk, the tree will struggle or die. Keep it at the same level it was in the pot.</u>

Layer 2: The Mid layer (Shrubs and Perennial Plants)

These are the plants that produce year after year with no need to be replanted. They fill the space under your trees and give you consistent harvests with minimal work.

This layer is where you get your greens, herbs, and perennial vegetables.

Moringa

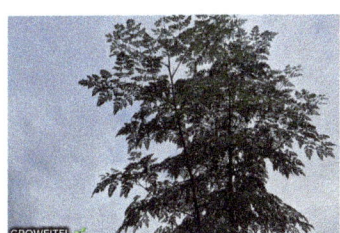

Moringa Tree

Zones: 9-11 (dies back in freezes but regrows from roots in zone 9)

This is your superfood. The leaves contain protein, vitamins, and minerals. People call it the "miracle tree" for a reason.

Planting: Full sun. Space 6-10 feet apart.

Care: Moringa grows fast. I mean, really fast. In Florida's heat, it can grow 10 to 15 feet in a year. Cut it back to 3-4 feet every few months to keep it bushy and encourage new leaf growth.

Harvesting: Pick the young leaves and tender stems. You can eat them raw in salads, cooked like spinach, or dried for tea.

When it produces: year-round in South Florida. Spring through fall in North Florida.

Beginner tip: Moringa is nearly impossible to kill. If you cut it back too hard, it regrows. If it freezes, it comes back from the roots. Just plant it and harvest constantly.

Katuk (Sauropus androgynus)

Zones: 8-11

Katuk is a leafy green that tastes like peas. It's popular in Southeast Asian cuisine and grows incredibly well in Florida.

Planting: Partial shade to full sun. Space 3 to 4 feet apart.

Care: Minimal. It handles heat, humidity, and shade. Prune it to keep it bushy.

Harvesting: Pick the leaves and tender tips. Eat them raw or cooked.

When it produces year-round.

Beginner tip: Katuk is one of those plants you plant once and forget about. It just keeps producing. And it actually grows better in partial shade, so it's perfect under your fruit trees.

Longevity Spinach (Gynura procumbens)

Zones: 9-11

Another medicinal green that's easy to grow and highly productive.

Planting: Partial shade. Space 2 to 3 feet apart.

Care: Keep it moist. It loves humidity.

Harvesting: Pick the leaves for salads or tea. It has a slightly bitter taste.

When it produces year-round.

Beginner tip: Longevity spinach spreads by rooting at the nodes. One plant becomes many. Give it space, ***or keep it contained.***

Cranberry Hibiscus (Hibiscus acetosella)

Zones: 8-11

Beautiful plant with deep red leaves that are edible and high in antioxidants.

Planting: Full sun to partial shade. Space 3 to 4 feet apart.

Care: Tolerates heat and humidity. Prune to keep it compact.

Harvesting: Pick the leaves for salads or cook them like greens. They have a tangy, lemony flavor.

When it produces: year-round.

Beginner tip: This plant is gorgeous. Use it as an ornamental that also feeds you. The leaves taste best when they're young and tender.

Lemongrass

Zones: 8-11

Lemongrass is a tropical grass that's used in cooking and tea. It grows in clumps and spreads.

Planting: Full sun. Space 2 to 3 feet apart.

Care: Minimal. It loves heat and sun. Divide the clumps every year or two.

Harvesting: Cut the stalks at the base. Use the white part for cooking. The green tops make great tea.

When it produces year-round.

Beginner tip: Start with one plant. In a year, you'll have a clump big enough to divide into 5-10 plants. Spread them around your property or give them to friends.

Turmeric and Ginger

Zones: 8-11

Both grow from rhizomes (thick underground stems). They're tropical plants that love Florida's heat and humidity.

Planting: Partial shade to full sun. Plant the rhizomes 2-3 inches deep in spring.

Care: Keep them watered during the growing season. Mulch heavily.

Harvesting: Dig them up in fall or winter after the leaves die back. Replant some, eat the rest.

When they produce: Plant in spring, harvest in fall/winter.

Beginner tip: Fresh turmeric and ginger are incredibly expensive at the store. Growing your own is a huge money-saver. Plus, they taste way better fresh than dried.

Rosemary

Zones: 8-10

Rosemary is a perennial herb that can handle Florida's heat if it has good drainage.

Planting: Full sun. Well-drained soil. Plant in a raised bed or container if your soil stays wet.

Care: Don't over-water. Rosemary prefers dry conditions.

Harvesting: Snip stems as needed. Use fresh or dried.

When it produces year-round.

Beginner tip: Rosemary struggles in Florida's wet season if the soil doesn't drain. Planting it in a container or raised bed solves this problem.

Pigeon Peas

Zones: 9-11

Pigeon peas are technically annuals, but they reseed themselves and act like perennials in Florida.

Planting: Full sun. Space 4 to 6 feet apart.

Care: Minimal. They fix nitrogen in the soil, so they actually improve your soil while growing.

Harvesting: Pick the green peas for cooking. Let some dry for storage.

When they produce summer through fall.

Beginner tip: Pigeon peas grow tall (6-10 feet) and provide shade for smaller plants. They're also a great chop-and-drop plant. Cut them back and leave the branches as mulch.

Layer 3: The Ground Cover (Annuals and Root Crops)

This is where you rotate crops based on the season. This layer changes throughout the year, and understanding what to plant when is the key to year-round food production.

Let me break this down by season, with specific planting windows and detailed instructions.

Cool Season Planting Guide (October - March)

This is prime-time in Florida. It's perfect weather. The bugs are manageable. The plants thrive.

This is when you go all-in.

Tomatoes

Planting window: October - February (earlier is better)

Varieties for Florida:

- 'Celebrity': Disease-resistant, reliable
- 'Better Boy': Large fruit, consistent producer
- 'Cherry tomatoes' (any variety): Easier to grow than large slicers
- 'Florida 91': Bred specifically for Florida's climate

How to plant:

1. Start with transplants, not seeds (unless you're experienced)
2. Plant them deep, burying 2/3 of the stem. This creates more roots.
3. Space them 2 to 3 feet apart.
4. Stake them immediately. Florida storms will knock them over otherwise.

Care:

- Water consistently. Tomatoes crack if they get inconsistent watering.
- Mulch heavily to keep moisture even.
- Fertilize every 2-3 weeks with a balanced organic fertilizer.

Harvesting: 60-85 days from transplant, depending on the variety.

Common problems:

- Hornworms: Large green caterpillars that eat leaves. Hand-pick them.
- Early blight: Brown spots on lower leaves. Remove affected leaves and mulch to prevent soil splash.
- Blossom end rot: Black spots on the bottom of fruit. Caused by inconsistent watering.

Beginner tip: Cherry tomatoes are way easier than large tomatoes in Florida. Start there.

Peppers

Planting window: October - February

Varieties for Florida:

- Bell peppers: 'California Wonder', 'Keystone Resistant Giant'

- Hot peppers: Any variety works; they love Florida's heat

How to plant:

1. Start with transplants.
2. Space 18 to 24 inches apart.
3. Plant at the same depth they were in the pot.

Care:

- Peppers are easier than tomatoes. Less water, less fuss.
- Fertilize monthly.
- Mulch to keep roots cool.

Harvesting: 60-90 days from transplant.

Beginner tip: Hot peppers handle Florida's summer better than sweet peppers. If you want peppers year-round, focus on hot varieties.

Lettuce and Salad Greens

Planting window: October - March

Varieties for Florida:

- Loose-leaf lettuce (not head lettuce): 'Black Seeded Simpson', 'Oak Leaf', 'Red Sails'
- Arugula: Grows fast, peppery flavor
- Spinach: 'Bloomsdale', 'Space'

How to plant:

1. Direct seed into garden beds or containers.
2. Scatter seeds and cover lightly with soil.
3. Keep soil moist until germination (5-10 days).

Care:

- Lettuce is shallow-rooted. Water frequently but lightly.

Harvest the outer leaves and let the plant continue to grow.

Harvesting: 30-45 days from seed.

Beginner tip: Succession plant every 2-3 weeks for continuous harvests.

Kale, Collards, Chard

Planting window: October - February

Varieties for Florida:

- Kale: 'Lacinato' (Dinosaur Kale), 'Red Russian'

- Collards: 'Georgia Southern', 'Vates'

- Swiss Chard: 'Bright Lights', 'Fordhook Giant'

How to plant:

1. Start with transplants or direct seeding.

2. Space 18 to 24 inches apart.

Care:

- These are tough plants. They handle cold and light frost.

- Harvest outer leaves, letting the plant keep producing.

Harvesting: 50-70 days from seed/transplant.

Beginner tip: These plants keep producing for months. One planting can feed you all winter.

Broccoli and Cauliflower

Planting window: October - January (early planting is critical)

Varieties for Florida:

- Broccoli: 'Green Magic', 'Packman'

- Cauliflower: 'Snow Crown', 'Amazing'

How to plant:

1. Start with transplants.

2. Space 18 to 24 inches apart.

Care:

- They need consistent water and cool temperatures.

- Fertilize every 2-3 weeks.

Harvesting: 70-100 days from transplant.

Beginner tip: These are finicky in Florida. If you plant too late, they'll bolt in the spring heat. Get them in the ground by November.

Carrots

Planting window: October - January

Varieties for Florida:

- 'Danvers', 'Nantes', 'Chantenay'

How to plant:

1. Direct seed into loose, well-amended soil.

2. Carrots need loose soil to grow straight. If compacted soil is your issue, use containers or raised beds for your carrots.

Care:

- Keep soil moist until germination (10-14 days).

- Thin seedlings to 2-3 inches apart once they sprout.

Harvesting: 60-80 days from seed.

Beginner tip: Carrots are harder in Florida's sandy or clay soils. Containers work better for beginners.

Beets

Planting window: October - February

Varieties for Florida:

- 'Detroit Dark Red', 'Golden Beet'

How to plant:

1. Direct seeding.

2. Each seed is actually a cluster, so you'll need to thin them .

Care:

- Keep the soil moist.

- Thin to 3-4 inches apart.

Harvesting: 50-70 days from seed.

Beginner tip: You can eat both the roots and the greens. Double harvest.

Radishes

Planting window: October - March

Varieties for Florida:

- 'Cherry Belle', 'French Breakfast', 'Watermelon Radish'

How to plant:

1. Direct seeding.

2. Space 1 to 2 inches apart.

Care:

- Radishes are fast.

- Keep the soil moist.

Harvesting: 25-30 days from seed.

Beginner tip: Radishes are a great confidence builder for beginners. They grow fast and are hard to mess up.

Peas

Planting window: October - February

Varieties for Florida:

- Sugar snap peas: 'Sugar Ann', 'Super Sugar Snap'

- Snow peas: 'Oregon Sugar Pod'

How to plant:

1. Direct seeding.

2. Provide a trellis for them to climb.

Care:

- Peas like cool weather. Plant early.

- Keep the soil moist.

Harvesting: 60-70 days from seed.

Beginner tip: Peas struggle in Florida's heat. Get them in the ground by November at the latest.

Strawberries

Planting window: October - November

Varieties for Florida:

- 'Florida Radiance', 'Sweet Charlie', 'Festival'

How to plant:

1. Buy bare-root plants or transplants.

2. Plant in raised beds or containers for better drainage.

3. Space 12 inches apart.

Care:

- Strawberries need consistent water and fertilizer.

- Mulch with straw to keep berries clean.

Harvesting: December - April.

Beginner tip: Strawberries are perennial in Florida but perform best if replanted every 2-3 years.

Herbs: Cilantro, Parsley, Dill

Planting window: October - February

How to plant:

1. Direct seed or transplant.

2. Space 6 to 8 inches apart.

Care:

- These herbs love cool weather.

- Harvest frequently to keep them from bolting.

Beginner tip: Cilantro bolts (goes to seed) fast in Florida. Succession planting every 2-3 weeks.

Warm-Season Planting Guide (April - September)

This is survival mode because the temperature is rising. The bugs are relentless. The afternoon storm floods everything.

But you can still grow food. You just need to pick the right plants.

Sweet Potatoes

Planting window: March - July

Varieties for Florida:

- 'Beauregard', 'Covington', 'Okinawan Purple'

How to plant:

1. Buy slips (rooted cuttings) or make your own from a sweet potato.

2. Plant in mounds or raised rows.

3. Space 12-18 inches apart.

Care:

- Sweet potatoes need space to sprawl. Give them room.

- Water regularly until established, then they're drought tolerant.

Harvesting: 90-120 days from planting. Dig them up in the fall.

Beginner tip: One slip can produce 5-10 pounds of sweet potatoes. This is a high-return crop.

Okra

Planting window: March - August

Varieties for Florida:

- 'Clemson Spineless', 'Burgundy', 'Emerald'

How to plant:

1. Direct seed after the soil warms up.

2. Space 12-18 inches apart.

Care:

- Okra loves heat. It thrives when everything else is struggling.

- Harvest every 2-3 days to keep it producing.

Harvesting: 50-60 days from seed.

Beginner tip: Pick the pods when they're 3-4 inches long. If you let them get too big, they get woody.

Southern Peas (Cowpeas)

Planting window: March - August

Varieties for Florida:

- 'Black-eyed peas', 'Crowder peas', 'Zipper peas'

How to plant:

1. Direct seeding.

2. Space 4-6 inches apart.

Care:

- These peas love heat and humidity.

- They fix nitrogen, so they improve your soil.

Harvesting: 60-90 days from seed.

Beginner tip: Let some pods dry on the plant for storage. You'll have seeds for next year and dried peas for cooking.

Eggplant

Planting window: March - August

Varieties for Florida:

- 'Black Beauty', 'Ichiban', 'Thai Long Green'

How to plant:

1. Start with transplants.

2. Space 24-36 inches apart.

Care:

- Eggplant handles heat well.
- Watch for flea beetles (small black bugs that eat holes in leaves).

Harvesting: 70-85 days from transplant.

Beginner tip: Harvest when the fruit is still shiny. Once it dulls, it's overripe.

Tropical Pumpkins and Squash

Planting window: March - July

Varieties for Florida:

- 'Seminole Pumpkin': Native to Florida, incredibly productive
- 'Calabaza': Cuban squash, loves heat

How to plant:

1. Direct seeding.
2. Give them tons of space. These vines spread 10 to 20 feet.

Care:

- Water consistently.
- Watch out for squash vine borers (they kill the vines from the inside).

Harvesting: 90-120 days from seed.

Beginner tip: Seminole pumpkin is nearly indestructible in Florida. It's the easiest squash you'll ever grow.

Cucumbers

Planting window: March - April, then again in August

How to plant:

1. Direct seed or transplant.
2. Provide a trellis.

Care:

- Cucumbers struggle in the peak heat of summer. Plant early or late.

- Keep them well-watered.

Harvesting: 50-70 days from seed.

Beginner tip: Powdery mildew (white powder on leaves) is common. Pick resistant varieties.

Beans

Planting window: March - April, then September

Varieties for Florida:

- Bush beans: 'Contender', 'Provider'
- Pole beans: 'Kentucky Wonder', 'Rattlesnake'

How to plant:

1. Direct seeding.
2. Pole beans need a trellis.

Care:

- Beans fix nitrogen in the soil.
- Pick regularly to keep them producing.

Harvesting: 50-60 days from seed.

Beginner tip: Bush beans are easier than pole beans for beginners.

Hot Peppers

Planting window: March - September

Varieties for Florida:

- 'Jalapeño', 'Serrano', 'Habanero', 'Thai Chili'

How to plant:

1. Transplant.
2. Space 18 to 24 inches apart.

Care:

- Hot peppers love Florida's heat.
- They'll produce year-round in South Florida.

Harvesting: 60-90 days from transplant.

Beginner tip: Hot peppers are way more productive than sweet peppers in Florida. If you like spice, grow these.

Herbs: Basil, Thai Basil, Oregano

Planting window: March - September

How to plant:

1. Transplant or direct-seed.
2. Space 12 inches apart.

Care:

- Basil loves heat and humidity.
- Pinch off flowers to keep it producing leaves.

Beginner tip: Thai basil handles Florida's summer better than sweet basil.

Building Soil in Florida's Sand

Let's talk about the biggest challenge in Florida gardening: the soil.

Or lack of it.

Most of Florida sits on sand. Pure, white, beach-quality sand. The kind you'd love to walk on barefoot but absolutely hate to garden in.

Sand drains too fast. It holds no nutrients. It bakes hard in the sun. And if you try to grow food in pure sand, you're going to fail.

So you need to build soil. And I mean actually build it, layer by layer, year after year.

Here's how.

Step 1: Mulch everything

This is non-negotiable in Florida.

Bare soil is dead soil. Florida sun bakes it. The rain washes it away. The nutrients leach out.

Mulch protects your soil. This helps to keep moisture in and keeps the temperature stable. It breaks down over time and adds organic matter. It suppresses weeds. And it feeds the soil life (bacteria, fungi, worms) that actually grow your plants.

In Florida, you need 3 to 4 inches of mulch around every plant, every bed, and every tree. All the time.

What to use:

- Wood chips: Free from tree services. Call local arborists and ask if they'll dump a load in your driveway.

- Leaves: Rake them up in the fall and spread them around your garden.

- Grass clippings: Use them in thin layers and let them dry first, or they'll mat and smell.

- Straw: Buy it from feed stores. Make sure it's straw (stems) and not hay (which has seeds).

How to apply:

- Spread it 3 to 4 inches thick.

- Keep it a few inches away from plant stems and tree trunks to avoid rot.

- Replenish it every few months as it breaks down.

Common mistake: People put down one inch of mulch and wonder why it doesn't work. You need thickness. Three to four inches minimum.

Step 2: Compost Constantly

Compost is how you turn garbage into gold.

Every kitchen scrap, every yard waste, every dead plant, every handful of weeds goes into the compost pile.

In Florida's heat, compost breaks down fast. If you turn it regularly and keep it moist, you can have finished compost in 2-3 months.

What goes in:

- Greens (high nitrogen): Kitchen scraps, grass clippings, coffee grounds, green plant material
- Browns (high carbon): Leaves, wood chips, cardboard, straw

The ratio: Aim for 2 parts brown to 1 part green.

How to build a pile:

1. Start with a layer of browns (leaves, straw).
2. Add a layer of greens (kitchen scraps, grass clippings).
3. Repeat.
4. Keep it moist (like a wrung-out sponge).
5. Turn it every week or two to add air.

Where to use it:

- Around trees
- In garden beds
- Mixed into planting holes
- As a top dressing on any plant

Beginner tip: You can't mess up compost. Even if you ignore it, it'll eventually break down. The more you tend it, the faster it works.

Step 3: Use cover crops

When you finish your cool-season beds in spring, don't leave them empty.

Plant a cover crop.

Cover crops are plants you grow not to eat but to improve the soil. They add organic matter, fix nitrogen, choke out weeds, and prevent erosion.

Best cover crops for Florida summers:

- Sunn hemp: Grows fast, fixes nitrogen, produces tons of biomass
- Cowpeas: Edible and improves soil
- Buckwheat: Quick-growing, attracts pollinators

How to use them:

1. Broadcast seeds over your empty bed.
2. Water them in.
3. Let them grow for 6 to 8 weeks.
4. Chop them down before they go to seed.
5. Leave the plant material on the soil as mulch.

Within a few weeks, it'll break down and feed your next crop.

Step 4: Stop tilling

Tilling is the worst thing you can do to Florida soil.

Every time you till, you:

- Kill the soil life (bacteria, fungi, worms)
- Burn up organic matter
- Destroy soil structure
- Bring weed seeds to the surface

Instead, build on top of the soil.

Add compost. Add mulch. Let the plant roots and soil life do the work of breaking up compacted soil.

This is called no-till gardening, and it's the best approach for Florida.

Step 5: Add amendments carefully

Florida soil is typically low in organic matter and certain nutrients.

But don't just throw fertilizer at it. That's expensive and short-term.

Instead, focus on long-term soil building:

- Compost: Adds organic matter and slow-release nutrients
- Worm castings: Rich in nutrients and beneficial microbes
- Bone meal: Adds phosphorus for root development
- Greensand: Adds potassium and trace minerals
- Azomite: Rock dust with trace minerals

For most plants, a good layer of compost twice a year is all you need.

For heavy feeders (tomatoes, peppers, squash), add a balanced organic fertilizer monthly during the growing season.

Beginner tip: Don't overthink it. Compost and mulch will solve 80% of your soil problems.

Water Management in Florida

Florida water is a study in extremes.

In the dry season, you can go weeks without rain. In the wet season, you can get 3 inches in an hour.

Learning to manage both is critical.

Dry Season Watering

Your established trees and perennials can usually handle dry spells once their roots are deep. But young plants and annuals need consistent watering.

How to water effectively:

- Use drip irrigation or soaker hoses. They're way more efficient than sprinklers.

- Water deeply, but less often. This trains roots to grow deep.

- Water in the early morning. Plants have all day to dry off, and you lose less to evaporation.

How much to water:

- Newly planted trees: 2-3 times per week for the first year

- Established trees: Rarely (let rain do the work)

- Vegetables and annuals: Daily in containers, every 2-3 days in the ground

- Perennials: Once or twice a week

Signs you're over-watering:

- Yellow leaves

- Wilting even when the soil is wet

- Fungal growth

- Root rot

Signs you're under-watering:

- Wilting in the heat of the day

- Dry, cracked soil

- Slow growth

- Fruit drop

Beginner tip: Stick your finger in the soil. If it's dry 2 inches down, water. If it's moist, wait.

Wet Season Management

If your soil doesn't drain well, the wet season will drown your plants.

Signs of poor drainage:

- Water standing in the garden after rain

- Soil that stays soggy for days

- Plants wilting even in wet soil (because roots can't breathe)

Solutions:

- Plant on mounds or raised beds. Even 8-12 inches of height makes an enormous difference.

- Add compost and mulch to improve soil structure.

- Choose plants that tolerate wet feet: sweet potatoes, taro, cranberry hibiscus, katuk, longevity spinach.

- Dig shallow drainage Swales to move water away from planting areas.

If you've got low spots that flood every summer, don't fight it. Turn it into a feature. Plant something that loves water.

Beginner tip: Raised beds solve most drainage problems in Florida.

Dealing with Florida Pests

Let's be real. Florida bugs are no joke.

We've got aphids, whiteflies, caterpillars, mealybugs, spider mites, thrips, leaf miners, stink bugs, and about a thousand other things trying to eat your food before you do.

You will not eliminate pests. That's not the goal. The goal is to keep them at manageable levels so you still get a harvest.

Here's the hierarchy of pest control, from least to most intervention.

Level 1: Prevention

Healthy soil = healthy plants = plants that can fight off pests.

This is the foundation. Weak plants attract pests. Strong plants resist them.

How to build healthy plants:

- Feed the soil with compost and mulch.
- Water consistently.
- Choose varieties suited to Florida's climate.
- Don't overcrowd plants (air circulation prevents disease and pests).

Diversity is your friend. A garden with 20 different plants is way more resilient than a garden with just tomatoes. Pests that specialize in one crop can't wipe you out if you're growing a mix.

Plant flowering herbs and flowers to attract beneficial insects (ladybugs, lacewings, parasitic wasps) that eat pests.

Good plants for attracting beneficial insects:

- Basil
- Dill

- Fennel
- Marigolds
- Zinnias

Level 2: Manual Removal

This is old-school pest control. You go out with your hands or a bucket and remove the pests.

Hand-picking works for:
- Caterpillars (hornworms, cabbage worms)
- Beetles
- Snails and slugs
- Egg clusters on leaves

Spraying with a hose works for:
- Aphids (blast them off with water)
- Spider mites
- Light infestations of soft-bodied insects

Check your plants every few days. Catching pests early makes a vast difference.

Level 3: Organic Sprays

When manual removal isn't enough, you can use organic sprays.

Neem oil:
- Works on soft-bodied insects (aphids, whiteflies, mealybugs)
- Mix 2 tablespoons per gallon of water
- Spray early morning or late evening (not in full sun)

BT (Bacillus thuringiensis):
- Biological control of caterpillars
- Safe for beneficial insects
- Spray on leaves where caterpillars are feeding

Insecticidal soap:

- Works on aphids, whiteflies, spider mites

- Spray directly on insects

- Repeat every few days

Diatomaceous earth:

- Sprinkle around plants to deter slugs, snails, and crawling insects

- Reapply after rain

Beginner tip: Rotate your sprays. Pests build resistance if you use the same thing over and over.

Level 4: Accept Some Loss

You will not save every leaf. Some damage is okay.

A plant can lose 20-30% of its leaves and still produce fine.

The goal is a harvest, not perfection.

If pests completely overwhelm a plant, pull it out and compost it (or throw it away if it's diseased). Don't waste energy fighting a losing battle.

Common Florida Pests and How to Deal with Them

Aphids:

- Small, soft-bodied insects that cluster on fresh growth

- Spray with water or neem oil

- Attract ladybugs (they eat aphids)

Whiteflies:

- Tiny white flying insects that live under leaves

- Yellow sticky traps

- Neem oil

- Insecticidal soap

Hornworms:

- Large green caterpillars that eat tomato and pepper leaves

- Hand-pick them (they're easy to spot)
- BT spray

Squash vine borers:
- Larvae that tunnel into squash and pumpkin stems
- Hard to control once inside
- Prevention: Plant early or late to avoid the peak season
- Row covers until flowering

Leaf miners:
- Larvae that tunnel between leaf layers, leaving squiggly lines
- Remove affected leaves
- Won't kill the plant, just cosmetic

Stink bugs:
- Shield-shaped bugs that suck plant juices
- Hand-pick them
- Trap crops (plant something they like more, like mustard greens)

Spider mites:
- Tiny mites that cause stippling (tiny white dots) on leaves
- Spray with water
- Neem oil

Beginner tip: Most pest problems are temporary. The population spikes, then beneficial insects show up and eat them. Be patient.

Dealing with Florida Storms and Hurricanes

Florida storms are a fact of life. From afternoon thunderstorms to full-blown hurricanes, your garden will take a beating at some point.

Here's how to minimize damage.

Before the Storm

Stake everything. Tomatoes, peppers, young trees, anything that can blow over.

Harvest what you can. If a hurricane is coming and your tomatoes are close to ripe, pick them. They'll ripen inside.

Mulch heavily. This prevents soil erosion during heavy rains.

Prune dead branches from trees. They'll become projectiles in high winds.

For potted plants, move them to a sheltered spot or lay them on their sides.

After the Storm

Check for broken branches and prune them cleanly.

Stand up plants that got knocked over. They'll usually recover.

Check for standing water. Don't walk on flooded beds, as you'll compact the soil. Let them drain first.

Replant what you lost. Seeds are cheap. Your time is valuable, but starting over is part of gardening in Florida.

***Beginner tip: Don't plant expensive, fragile plants during hurricane season (June-November). Save them for* the fall.**

Your First-Year Timeline

Let me walk you through what your first year could look like if you start right now, month by month.

This is a realistic timeline for someone starting from scratch.

Month 1 (January):

- Plant 2-3 fruit trees (mango, avocado, citrus, loquat, or papaya)

- Start a compost pile (even if it's just a pile in the yard's corner)

- Plant cool-season annuals: tomatoes, peppers, greens, radishes

- Mulch everything heavily (3-4 inches)

What you're learning: How to plant. Where the sun hits. How much water plants need.

Month 2 (February):
- Add perennials: moringa, katuk, lemongrass
- Succession planting: more greens and radishes
- Observe your space: Where does water collect? Where's it dry?

What you're learning: Plant spacing. Watering schedules. How fast things grow in Florida.

Month 3 (March):
- Harvest your first greens and radishes (this is exciting!)
- Plant sweet potato slips
- Transition to summer crops: okra, southern peas
- Start thinking about the wet season strategy

What you're learning: The joy of harvesting. What worked, what didn't.

Month 4-5 (April-May):
- First tomato and pepper harvests (if you planted early enough)
- Summer heat kicks in
- Focus on mulching and watering
- Let your cool-season beds rest or plant cover crops

What you're learning: Florida heat is real. Not everything survives the summer.

Months 6-8 (June-August):
- Wet season survival mode
- Harvest okra, southern peas, herbs
- Observe which spots flood, which stay dry
- Your trees are growing (slowly, but they're growing)

What you're learning: patience. Some seasons are about maintenance, not production.

Month 9 (September):

- Start planning the cool season again
- Order seeds and seedlings
- Prepare beds with compost
- Clean up storm damage if needed

What you're learning: Planning makes everything easier.

Month 10-11 (October-November):

- Plant cool-season crops again
- This time you know what worked last year
- Harvest sweet potatoes from the spring planting
- Your trees have grown significantly

What you're learning: You're not a beginner anymore. You're a gardener.

Month 12 (December):

- Harvesting greens, radishes, early tomatoes
- First citrus fruits ripen
- Your garden has become a system
- You're not buying as many groceries

What you're learning: This works. And it's worth it.

That's one year.

In year two, your trees are bigger. Your perennials have become established. You know what works in your specific space. You're not guessing anymore.

By year three, you're harvesting fruit from trees. Your food forest is feeding you. And you're teaching other people how to do it.

The 80/20 of Florida food growing

If you're feeling overwhelmed, focus here.

These seven things will give you 80% of the results with 20% of the effort.

1. Plant 3-5 fruit trees now.

Even if you do nothing else, plant trees. Mango, avocado, citrus, loquat, papaya. They take years to produce, so the sooner you plant, the sooner you eat.

2. Grow moringa, katuk, and lemongrass as perennial greens.

Plant them once and harvest forever. These three alone can provide a significant amount of your greens year-round.

3. Go heavy on cool-season annuals (October-March).

This is Florida's money season. Load up on tomatoes, peppers, greens, and root crops. This is when you grow the bulk of your food.

4. Plant sweet potatoes and okra for the summer.

These two crops thrive in Florida's heat. They're your summer staples, while everything else struggles.

5. Mulch everything, all the time.

Three to four inches, constantly replenished. This single practice will save you more time, water, and frustration than anything else.

6. Compost your scraps.

Turn garbage into soil. Every kitchen scrap, every yard waste, every dead plant goes in the pile. Use the finished compost everywhere.

7. Water consistently, but not obsessively.

Deep watering 2-3 times per week is better than shallow watering every day. Train roots to go deep.

That's it. That's the core.

Everything else is an optimization.

Common Mistakes Florida Gardeners Make

Let me save you some pain by pointing out the mistakes I see all the time.

Mistake 1: Planting tomatoes in June.

Tomatoes are a cool-season crop in Florida. Plant them October through February. If you try to grow them in summer, they'll get diseases, struggle with the heat, and break your heart.

Mistake 2: Not mulching.

I can't stress this enough. Florida soil without mulch dries out in hours. Your plants cook. Your water bill skyrockets. Mulch is non-negotiable.

Mistake 3: Fighting summer instead of working with it.

Summer is for sweet potatoes, okra, and letting your trees grow. Stop trying to force cool-season crops in the heat. It won't work.

Mistake 4: Planting trees too close together.

That cute little mango tree in a 3-gallon pot will be 30 feet wide in five years. Give it space. Don't crowd your trees. They need room to grow.

Mistake 5: Overwatering.

More plants die from over-watering than under-watering in Florida. Stick your finger into the soil. If it's wet, don't water it.

Mistake 6: Giving up after one failure.

You're going to kill the plants. Everyone does. A plant dies? That's compost. Learn from it and try again. You learn to garden by doing, not by reading.

Mistake 7: Ignoring your soil.

You can't grow food in pure sand. Build your soil with compost and mulch. This takes time, but it's the foundation of everything.

Your Year-Round Harvest Calendar

Here's what you should harvest each month in a well-established Florida food forest.

This is your goal. In year one, you'll have some of this. Year three, you'll have most of it.

January:
- Greens (lettuce, kale, collards)
- Radishes
- Carrots
- Citrus (oranges, grapefruits, tangerines)
- Herbs (cilantro, parsley)

February:
- Tomatoes (early varieties)
- Peppers
- Broccoli
- Cauliflower
- Strawberries
- Citrus

March:
- Tomatoes (peak harvest)
- Peppers
- Greens
- Peas
- Citrus
- Loquats

April:
- Late tomatoes
- Peppers
- Mulberries
- Loquats

- Early mangoes (South Florida)

May:
- Mangoes
- Avocados
- Papayas

June:
- Mangoes (peak)
- Avocados
- Papayas
- Okra
- Southern peas

July:
- Mangoes (late varieties)
- Papayas
- Okra
- Southern peas
- Eggplant

August:
- Papayas
- Okra
- Southern peas
- Eggplant
- Herbs (basil, oregano)

September:
- Papayas
- Sweet potatoes (early harvest)
- Okra

- Peppers (if they survived the summer)

October:
- Sweet potatoes
- Papayas
- Early fall greens
- Early radishes

November:
- Greens
- Radishes
- Sweet potatoes
- Papayas
- Early tomatoes

December:
- Greens
- Radishes
- Herbs
- Early citrus
- Early tomatoes

Every single month, something is ready.

That's a year-round food forest.

This chapter pays for the book

I told you this chapter would pay for itself, and I meant it.

If you implement even half of what's here, you'll save hundreds of dollars on groceries in the first year. Thousands over five years.

A bag of organic greens at the store costs $5. You can grow $50 worth of greens from a $3 pack of seeds.

A mango tree costs $30 to $50. Once it produces, it'll give you hundreds of dollars worth of fruit every year. For decades.

Sweet potatoes cost $2 to $3 per pound at the store. One slip (which costs $1) can produce 5-10 pounds of potatoes.

Tomatoes in winter cost $4 to $5 per pound in Florida. You can grow 20 pounds from a $3 plant.

The math is absurd. Growing food saves money.

But more than that, you'll have security. Knowledge. Skills that last.

You'll know how to feed your family no matter what's happening in the world.

You'll know what's in your food. You'll know it's not sprayed with chemicals you can't pronounce.

You'll teach your kids that food doesn't come from a store. It comes from the ground.

And you'll have something to pass down. A food forest that keeps giving long after you're gone.

So go back through this chapter. Mark it up. Dog-ear the pages. Take notes in the margins.

Then get to work.

Because this isn't theory. This is the blueprint.

Everything you need to build a year-round food forest in Florida is right here.

Grow the plants. Identify the times when you should plant them. The techniques to make them thrive. The solutions to every problem you'll face.

I've given you everything I know.

Now it's up to you to plant it.

Get your hands in the dirt. Make mistakes. Learn. Adjust. Keep going.

And a year from now, when you're eating tomatoes in January and mangoes in June and sweet potatoes in October, you'll look back and realize this was the chapter that changed everything.

This was the chapter that paid for itself a hundred times over.

This was the chapter that gave you your freedom back.

Now go build it.

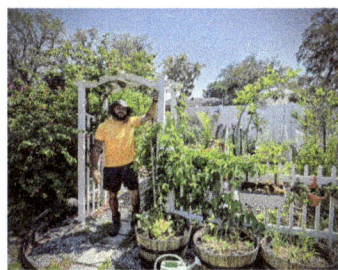

Jermaine is standing in front of one of his backyard garden areas.

Chapter 7

MEDICINAL HERBS

A Critical Note Before We Begin

Before we go any further, let me be absolutely clear about something.

I'm not a doctor. Medical advice is not something I can provide. Diagnosing, treating, or prescribing for your health conditions is beyond my qualifications.

This chapter does not contain any medical advice. The care of a qualified healthcare provider is irreplaceable by anything here. A professional must guide the use of anything here to treat serious illness.

Education is what this is. We can draw inspiration from this. Here, you'll find a look at my life, my experiences, and my ancestors' legacy.

But herbs are powerful. And powerful things demand respect.

Interacting with medications is something they can do. They can affect existing health conditions. They can cause allergic reactions. And yes, they can cause harm if used incorrectly or in excess.

If you are pregnant, nursing, taking any medications, or dealing with any health condition, chronic or acute, you must talk with a qualified healthcare provider before using any of these herbs.

Before stopping prescribed medication, you must speak with your doctor. Do not use herbs to replace professional medical care for serious conditions. Do not assume that because something is "natural," it's automatically safe.

Your health is too important to take risks with.

Now, with that said, let me share what I've learned. Because there is actual power here. Real wisdom. Generations have practiced real healing.

But it starts with respect. For the plants. For your body. And for the knowledge that came before us.

Let's begin.

From Fruit to Medicine

When I first started gardening, my obsession was fruit.

I wanted mangoes dripping from the branches. Avocados the size of footballs. Guavas so sweet the kids could eat until their hands were sticky and their shirts stained with juice.

That was the dream. A backyard fruit stand. A tropical paradise.

But there came a moment, somewhere in the middle of all that planting and harvesting, when I realized my backyard could be more than that.

It could be a medicine cabinet. A pharmacy without a waiting line. A place where healing grew right alongside the food.

That discovery changed everything.

I fell hard for medicinal herbs. They weren't quiet little plants sitting in the background anymore. They became alive with purpose, woven into our daily lives in ways I never expected.

My wife and I drink herbal tea every single day. Sometimes two or three times. One cup eases stress. Another supports healthy blood pressure. Another strengthens the immune system or addresses inflammation.

These herbs aren't trends we picked up on Instagram or read about in some wellness blog. They're traditions. My wife's family and my family have passed down these practices through generations.

My in-laws came from Haiti, where herbs weren't "alternative medicine." They were the first response.

Fever? Tea.

Stomach ache? Tea.

Infection? Tea.

My wife inherited that wisdom and has been teaching me one cup at a time. Showing me which leaves to pick. How long to steep them? What combinations work together?

And my mom? She carries the same torch.

Every morning, without fail, she brews her moringa tea. Sometimes she adds ginger or cinnamon. Sometimes she drinks it plain. But she never skips it.

And I believe deeply that this daily ritual is one reason she's still so sharp at her age. Still chasing her fourteen grandchildren around the yard. Still full of energy and life.

That's not luck. That's lifestyle.

The Chorus of Voices

Over the years, I've spoken to hundreds of people face-to-face and replied to thousands of comments on my YouTube channel, @GrowFitFL.

And the stories poured in.

People tell me about their grandmothers' remedies. Their uncle's secret tea. The plant their mother grew in the backyard that kept the family healthy when money was tight and doctors were far away.

What amazes me is how often the same plants show up in these stories.

No matter if it's someone in Florida, Georgia, Jamaica, Haiti, Puerto Rico, or halfway across the world, they tell me about the same herbs.

Moringa. Ginger. Cinnamon. Turmeric. Anamu. Lemongrass. soursop. Ashwagandha.

These are the heavy hitters. The plants people swear by. The ones that kept showing up in story after story, voice after voice, generation after generation.

And when you hear the same chorus long enough, you stop questioning. You plant.

I planted them all. In abundance.

Because if that many people, across that many cultures, over that many generations, are all saying the same thing, there's something real there.

Something worth paying attention to.

The Stories That Changed My Mind

Let me share some of these voices with you. Because they're not my stories to own. They belong to the people who lived them.

A man in Ocala wrote me that stress had broken him down after he lost his job. His immune system had failed. He was getting sick constantly. Couldn't sleep. Couldn't focus.

Someone told him about moringa.

He planted six trees in his backyard. Started drying the leaves for tea. Drank a cup every morning.

Within weeks, he said he felt like a new man. The brain fog lifted. The constant cold stopped. He had energy again.

Now, years later, he still has those six trees. Prunes them seasonally. Dries the leaves in batches. And swears moringa saved his life.

Then there was a subscriber from Miami who told me about her grandmother's ginger and honey tea.

Every time they got sick as kids, her grandmother would boil fresh ginger with lime and honey. Made them drink it hot, even when they complained about the burning.

She said it worked better than anything from the pharmacy. Faster. Stronger. And it never came with side effects or a long list of warnings.

I tested it myself when the flu hit me one winter. And I immediately understood why people have passed it down for generations.

Another woman wrote about cinnamon tea helping her husband's fasting blood sugar numbers.

He'd been struggling for years. Trying different diets. Different medications. Nothing seemed to work consistently.

Then someone told him to try cinnamon bark tea every night before bed.

He laughed at first. Said, "It's the only sweet thing that's ever helped my health."

But the numbers don't lie. His morning blood sugar readings dropped. His doctor noticed. And now he doesn't go a day without that tea.

These do not represent polished testimonials. They're not marketing slogans.

They're real people, some of them typing with tears in their eyes, telling me what got them through.

And that's when it hit me.

If all these voices were saying the same thing, I needed to do more than just listen. I needed to plant them all, right here in my Florida soil.

I didn't want to just read about their benefits or buy them dried and shipped from somewhere else.

I wanted to see them grow. Cut them fresh. Brew them myself. And pass them on to my family the way others had passed them down for generations.

What I Can and Cannot Promise You

I can't promise you that any one herb will fix everything. That's not how this works.

Herbs are not magic bullets. They're not miracle cures. They're tools. Powerful tools, but tools.

They work best as part of a bigger picture. Good food. Clean water. Movement. Rest. Stress management. Community. Purpose.

Herbs can't overcome a poor diet. You can't brew your way out of chronic sleep deprivation. You can't step away from the effects of untreated trauma.

But here's what I can promise you.

When you grow these plants, when you use them with respect and intention, you feel connected to something bigger than yourself.

You understand that healing doesn't always come from a bottle with a child-proof cap.

Sometimes it comes from your own soil. Your own hands. Your own daily rituals.

You see your backyard differently. Not just as decoration, but as provision. As protection. As a partnership with nature that has been healing people long before we existed, [continue sentence]

So before we dive into each herb, I want you to approach this with an open mind and a humble heart.

Do your research. Respect the power of these plants. Talk to your doctor if you have health conditions or take medication.

And ask yourself what it would mean for your family if the answers to stress, inflammation, or weakened immunity weren't a drive away, but a few steps outside your back door.

These are the herbs that shaped my garden, shaped my health, and changed the way I think about food and medicine.

Now, I want to share them with you.

The Essential Five: Where to Start

If you're just starting out and want a tight set of plants that thrive in Florida and actually deliver results, these are the five I lean on the most.

I grow over thirty-five medicinal herbs now, and I'm adding to my food forest almost every week. But these five form my foundation. The ones I come back to every single day.

Moringa: My Daily Multivitamin

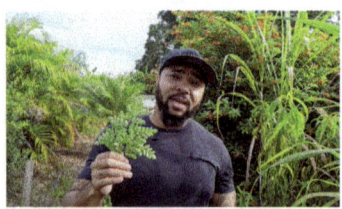

Jermaine holding some Moringa in his Food Forest

Scientific name: Moringa oleifera

This is my number one. My non-negotiables. My daily foundation.

Moringa is what I call my multivitamin tree. The leaves contain abundant vitamins A, C, E, calcium, potassium, protein, and many antioxidants.

Traditional uses: In tropical regions worldwide, moringa has been used to combat malnutrition, support lactation in nursing mothers, address inflammation, and boost overall vitality.

What the research says: Studies show moringa leaves contain high levels of nutrients and bioactive compounds with antioxidant and anti-inflammatory properties. Some research suggests moringa can help manage blood sugar and cholesterol levels, though researchers need more human studies.

How I use it: Fresh leaves in salads or cooked like spinach. Dried leaves for tea. Powdered leaves added to smoothies or food.

My mom drinks moringa tea every single morning with her Bible open beside her. As for years. And I believe it's one reason she's still sharp, still active, still chasing grandkids.

Growing moringa in Florida:

Zones: 9-11 (dies back in freezes but regrows from roots in zone 9)

Planting: Full sun. Space 6-10 feet apart. Plant from seed or cuttings.

Soil: Tolerates poor soil as long as it drains well. Moringa hates wet feet.

Growth: Fast. Insanely fast. In Florida's heat, a moringa tree can grow 10-15 feet in a year if conditions are right.

Pruning: This is critical. If you don't prune moringa, it'll grow into a tall, skinny tree with all the leaves at the top, out of reach.

Cut it back hard every 2-3 months to 3-4 feet. This forces it to bush out and produce tons of tender new growth at picking height.

Don't be gentle. Moringa responds to aggressive pruning by exploding with fresh shoots.

Harvesting: Pick the young leaves and tender stem tips. The younger, the better. Once leaves get large and tough, they're less palatable.

You can harvest year-round in South Florida. In North Florida, it'll die back in winter but regrow from the roots in spring.

Pests: pest-free. Occasionally aphids or caterpillars, but nothing serious.

Water: Water regularly when young. Once established, it's drought-tolerant.

Beginner tip: Moringa is nearly impossible to kill. If you cut it back too hard, it regrows. If it freezes, it comes back from the roots. Just plant it and start harvesting.

Safety and precautions:

- Considered safe when used as food

- Avoid root and bark (they contain compounds that can be toxic in large amounts)

- If pregnant or nursing, consult your healthcare provider before using medicinally

- May lower blood sugar, so monitor if you're diabetic or on blood sugar medications

- Start with small amounts to ensure you don't have digestive upset

Lemongrass (Fever Grass): The Foundation of Every Tea

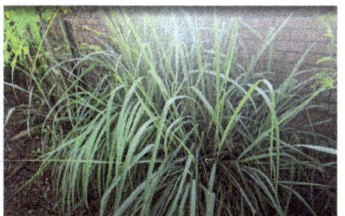

Lemongrass

Scientific name: Cymbopogon citratus

If you've watched my YouTube channel, you've seen me grab handfuls of lemongrass and chop it right into the pot.

It's the base note in almost every herbal tea I make. Not just for flavor, but because it ties everything together.

Traditional uses: Used across the tropics for digestive support, calming nerves, reducing fever, and relieving pain. In Caribbean culture, it's called "fever grass" and is the go-to remedy for colds and flu.

What the research says: Studies show lemongrass contains citral and other bioactive compounds with antimicrobial, anti-inflammatory, and antioxidant properties. Some research suggests benefits for anxiety, digestion, and pain relief.

How I use it: Fresh or dried in tea. I pack a good handful in there, boil it until the entire kitchen smells citrusy, then let it steep while I add other herbs.

Whether I'm making tea with soursop leaves, anamu, turmeric, or ginger, lemongrass smooths out the bitterness and makes the whole blend easier to drink.

To me, lemongrass isn't just another plant in the mix. It's the one that makes all the others feel like they belong together.

Growing lemongrass in Florida:

Zones: 8-11

Planting: Full sun. Plant divisions (clumps) 2-3 feet apart.

Soil: Tolerates a range of soils. Prefers rich, moist soil but handles Florida's sand if amended with compost.

Growth: Grows in clumps that expand. One plant becomes many.

Maintenance: Cut back to 6 inches once or twice a year to encourage fresh growth. Divide clumps every year or two and spread them around your property.

Harvesting: Cut stalks at the base. Use the white bottom part for cooking (Thai and Vietnamese cuisine). The green tops make excellent tea.

For tea, harvest the entire stalk, chop it into pieces, and boil it.

Pests: pest-free.

Water: Likes consistent moisture. Water regularly, especially during the dry season.

Beginner tip: Start with one plant. Within a year, you'll have a clump big enough to divide into 5-10 plants. It's one of the easiest herbs to propagate and share.

Safety and precautions:

- Safe when used in food and tea

- People should dilute essential oils for topical use because they are potent.

- Avoid high internal doses if pregnant

- Some people may experience skin irritation or dizziness with concentrated forms

- Start with moderate amounts in tea and observe how you feel

Turmeric: The Anti-Inflammatory Powerhouse

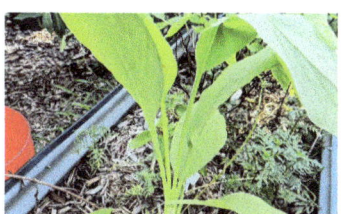
Turmeric

Scientific name: Curcuma longa

This is the herb that makes people cry. Not because it hurts, but because of what it gives back.

I remember a woman who wrote to me about her hands being so stiff from arthritis that she couldn't cook for her family anymore.

Opening jars was impossible. Chopping vegetables made her wince. Her loved ones couldn't enjoy her making dinner.

A neighbor gave her turmeric tea with black pepper (the pepper increases absorption).

After three weeks, she was opening jars again. Chopping vegetables. Cooking full meals.

She wrote to me through tears, saying she never thought she'd get that joy back.

Traditional uses: Used for thousands of years in Ayurvedic and traditional Chinese medicine for inflammation, digestive issues, skin conditions, and liver support.

They have extensively studied curcumin, the active compound in turmeric. Research shows strong anti-inflammatory and antioxidant effects. Studies suggest potential benefits for arthritis, metabolic syndrome, anxiety, and muscle soreness. Black pepper significantly increases its absorption.

How I use it: Fresh root grated into tea or golden milk (warm milk with turmeric, honey, and black pepper). Dried and powdered in food. Fresh slices in hot water as a simple tea.

My cousin swears by turmeric milk before bed. Says it takes the ache out of his bones and helps him sleep.

Growing turmeric in Florida:

Zones: 8-11

Planting: Plant rhizomes (the knobby root pieces) in spring, 2-3 inches deep, 8-12 inches apart. Partial shade to full sun.

Soil: Rich, well-amended soil. Turmeric is a heavy feeder. Add lots of compost.

Growth: The rhizomes sprout into tall, leafy plants (2-3 feet) that grow through spring and summer.

Harvesting: Dig up rhizomes in fall or early winter after the leaves die back. This is typically 8 to 10 months after planting.

Save some of the best rhizomes to replant. Use the rest fresh or dry them for storage.

Store fresh turmeric in the fridge for weeks or freeze it for months. To dry, slice thinly and dry in a dehydrator or low oven, then grind into powder.

Pests: pest-free.

Water: Keep soil consistently moist during the growing season.

Beginner tip: Fresh turmeric stains everything. Your hands, your cutting board, your clothes. Wear gloves when processing it. But that bright orange stain is a badge of honor.

Safety and precautions:

- Safe in food amounts
- High doses may cause digestive upset
- May increase bleeding risk; use caution if on blood thinners
- May lower blood sugar; monitor if diabetic
- Can interact with certain medications; check with your doctor
- Avoid high supplemental doses if pregnant
- The fresh root is less concentrated than supplements, making it safer for daily use

Aloe Vera: The First Aid Plant

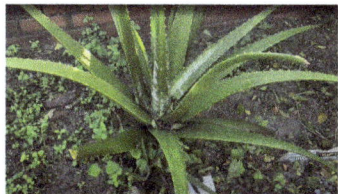

Aloe Vera

Scientific name: Aloe barbadensis miller

This one sits right by our house for a reason. It's the plant I go to for skin issues, burns, or cuts.

But I also use it internally, in tiny amounts and infrequently, when my digestive system needs a gentle reset.

Traditional uses: Used for thousands of years for skin healing, burns, wounds, and digestive support. People apply the gel topically.

What the research says: The gel is well-studied for skin healing, particularly for burns and wound healing. It has antimicrobial and anti-inflammatory properties. Using the latex requires extreme caution because it is a strong laxative.

How I use it: Topically for minor burns, cuts, and skin irritation. Occasionally, a small amount of inner gel (not the latex) in water for digestive support.

I keep multiple aloe plants around the property. Next to the kitchen door. One by the grill. One near the garden where the kids play.

Because when you need aloe, you need it now. Not ten minutes from now, after you go searching.

Growing aloe in Florida:

You can grow them in pots in zones 9-11 and bring them inside in colder zones.

Planting: Full sun to partial shade. Plant in well-draining soil or containers.

Soil: Must drain well. Aloe is a succulent and will rot in wet soil. Mix sand or perlite into your soil if needed.

Growth: Aloe grows in rosettes and produces "pups" (baby plants) around the base.

Maintenance: Remove dead leaves. Divide and replant pups as they form.

Harvesting: Cut outer leaves at the base. Let the yellow latex drain out (don't use this part internally). Fillet the leaf to extract the clear gel inside.

Pests: pest-free. Watch for mealybugs occasionally.

Water: Water sparingly. Aloe is drought-tolerant. More plants die from over-watering than under-watering.

Beginner tip: Aloe is one of the easiest plants to grow and propagate. One plant becomes dozens over a few years.

Safety and precautions:

- Topical gel is safe for most people
- Some people are allergic; test on a small area first
- The yellow latex just under the skin is a strong laxative and can cause cramping, diarrhea, and electrolyte imbalance
- Do not use latex internally if pregnant, nursing, or have digestive disorders
- Internal use of gel should be minimal and infrequent
- Never use latex internally without medical supervision
- Some medications interact with aloe; check with your doctor

Ashwagandha: The Stress Manager

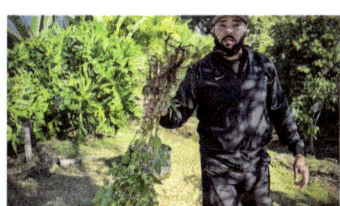

Harvesting Ashwagandha

Scientific name: Withania somnifera

This is the herb that came to me at exactly the right time. The one that still makes me pause and thank God.

After my father passed away , I was struggling. Grief sat heavy on my chest. Sleep was hard. Focus was impossible. I felt as if I were moving through the world underwater.

I spent night after night researching herbs, looking for something, anything, that might help.

I kept coming back to ashwagandha. An adaptogen used in Ayurvedic medicine for thousands of years to help the body manage stress and restore balance.

Then one afternoon, my wife came home holding a little packet. Ashwagandha seeds.

She did not know that was the very plant I'd been studying. No idea I'd spent hours reading about it. She just felt led to buy them.

I planted those seeds with shaking hands. Prayed over them. Watched them grow.

And that season reminded me of a truth I hold close: God always provides.

Praise God.

Traditional uses: Used in Ayurvedic medicine as a rejuvenating tonic, to combat stress and fatigue, support sleep, enhance vitality, and improve focus.

What the research says: Ashwagandha is one of the most studied adaptogen. Research shows it can reduce cortisol (stress hormone), improve sleep quality, reduce anxiety, enhance physical performance, and support cognitive function.

How I use it: Dried root powdered in tea or capsules. I take it in the evening as part of my wind-down routine.

Life doesn't slow down. But ashwagandha helps me manage it. Helps me find my rhythm. Helps me sleep when my mind won't stop.

Growing ashwagandha in Florida:

Zones: 8-11 (annual in most of Florida; may overwinter in zone 10)

Planting: Full sun. Plant seeds or transplants in the spring. Space 12 to 18 inches apart.

Soil: Well-draining soil. Ashwagandha doesn't like wet feet.

Growth: Grows into a small shrub (2-3 feet) with small flowers and red berries.

Harvesting: The roots are the medicinal part. Dig them up in the fall after the plant has grown for 6-8 months. The older the root, the more potent it is .

Wash, slice, and dry the roots. Grind into powder or use pieces for tea.

Pests: pest-free.

Water: Moderate watering. Don't over water.

Beginner tip: Ashwagandha is not as vigorous in Florida as some other herbs, but it's worth growing. If you struggle with it, you can always purchase the dried root from reputable sources.

Safety and precautions:

- Safe for most people in moderate doses

- Avoid if pregnant or breastfeeding (traditionally used to induce miscarriage)

- May interact with thyroid medications, sedatives, and immunosuppressants

- May lower blood sugar and blood pressure; monitor if on related medications

- Start with small doses and observe the effects

- Take breaks; don't use continuously for months without a break

- If you have autoimmune conditions, consult your doctor first

The Extended Medicine Cabinet: More Herbs Worth Knowing

These five are my foundation. But my garden holds so much more.

Let me walk you through some of the other powerful herbs, respect how they grow in Florida, and what you need to know about using them safely.

Soursop (Graviola)

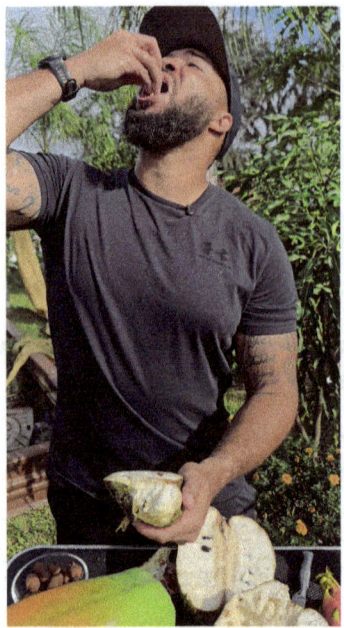

Eating Soursop straight from my tree

Scientific name: Annona muricata

Soursop is the plant people talk about with emotion in their voices.

A man once told me about his aunt battling cancer. The treatments left her weak, unable to eat, and constantly nauseated .

A neighbor brought her soursop leaves and told her to make tea.

She brewed it every night, sipping slowly. And for the first time in weeks, she could finish a small meal.

He said it didn't cure her. But it gave her quality of life when she needed it most. And to him, that was a miracle.

Another woman wrote about her grandmother in Puerto Rico, who grew a massive soursop tree behind her house.

Whenever someone in the family was sick, she'd make tea from the leaves, saying, "This is God's gift."

That tree became the family's pharmacy. And years later, even after the grandmother passed, the children kept planting soursop in her honor.

For them, it wasn't just about health. It was about memory. About carrying forward the strength of the one who raised them.

Traditional uses: People throughout the Caribbean and Central America use soursop leaves for infections, inflammation, pain, hypertension, and to support the body during illness.

What the research says: Lab studies show soursop contains compounds called acetogenins with potential anti-cancer, antimicrobial, and antioxidant properties. However, humans have limited clinical evidence. There are also safety concerns with long-term or high-dose use.

The fruit: sweet, custard-like, delicious. Kids love it frozen, blended, or eaten fresh.

The leaves: This is where the medicinal use focuses.

Growing soursop in Florida:

Zones: 10-11 (very sensitive to cold; in zone 9B only with heavy protection)

Planting: Full sun. Rich, well-draining soil. Space 15 to 20 feet apart.

Cold sensitivity: This is the challenge. Temperatures below 32°F can kill soursop trees.

In South Florida, they do well. In Central and North Florida, you will need to protect them in winter or grow them in large containers that you can move.

Growth: Slow to moderate. Trees can reach 15 to 20 feet at maturity.

Harvesting fruit: The fruit is ready when it's slightly soft and the skin is yellowish-green. Pick before it gets too soft or it'll split.

Harvesting leaves: Pick mature, green leaves. Dry in shade. Store in airtight containers.

Pests: Watch for scale and mealybugs.

Water: Regular watering, especially when young.

Beginner tip: Even in South Florida, be prepared to wrap or cover your soursop tree during cold snaps. People go to great lengths to protect these trees because they know what they mean.

Safety and precautions:

- The fruit is safe to eat
- Do not consume the seeds (they contain toxic compounds)
- Long-term or high-dose use of leaf tea raises concerns about neurotoxicity
- Researchers have linked compounds called annonaceous acetogenins, particularly annonacin, to neurological issues in animal studies.
- Use leaf tea in moderation and not continuously
- Avoid if pregnant or nursing
- May lower blood pressure and blood sugar; monitor if on related medications
- If you have Parkinson's disease or movement disorders, avoid soursop
- This is not a substitute for cancer treatment; always work with your oncologist

Anamu (Guinea Hen Weed)

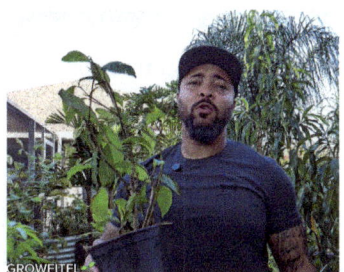

Jermaine holding Guinea Hen Weed Plant

Scientific name: Petiveria alliacea

This is probably my favorite herb to turn into tea. Every time I drink it, I feel like I've given my body one of the strongest forms of support I could.

The first time I came across anamu, I wasn't even looking for it. I'd been hearing about it for years from people from the islands.

Their parents and grandparents used it for everything from pain to "cleansing the body." I brushed it off at first.

But after hearing it again and again, I tracked some down.

The smell hit me before anything else. Strong, earthy, with a garlic-like punch that makes you believe it has power.

I planted it in my yard, and it surprised me with how tough it was. Florida storms didn't bother it. The heat didn't burn it. It just kept growing as if it belonged.

The first time I brewed it, I'll be honest, it wasn't a tea you sit back and savor. It was bitter. Pungent. Medicine.

And that was exactly the point.

Traditional uses: Used throughout the Caribbean and Central/South America for immune support, pain, infections, inflammation, and traditionally for tumors.

What the research says: Studies show antimicrobial, anti-inflammatory, and analgesic (pain-relieving) activity in laboratory and animal models. Some research on immune modulation and anti-cancer properties, but human data is very limited.

How I use it: Dried leaves in tea, often combined with lemongrass to balance the bitterness.

Growing anamu in Florida:

Zones: 9-11

Planting: Partial shade to full sun. Space 2 to 3 feet apart.

Soil: Well-draining. Tolerates poor soil.

Growth: Grows into a small shrub (1-3 feet). Spreads by underground runners, so it can become a colony.

Harvesting: Cut leaves and stems. Dry in shade. The whole plant has medicinal properties.

Pests: pest-free.

Water: Moderate. It's fairly drought-tolerant once established.

Beginner tip: Anamu has a strong smell (hence "garlic weed"). Plant it somewhere you won't be brushing against it constantly.

Safety and precautions:

- Avoid if pregnant or breastfeeding (traditionally used to induce menstruation and labor)

- May increase bleeding risk; avoid if on blood thinners

- May lower blood sugar; monitor if diabetic

- Can cause uterine contractions

- The smell can be very strong; some people find it off-putting
- Start with small amounts in tea
- This is a powerful herb; treat it with respect

Ginger

Scientific name: Zingiber officinale

A subscriber from Miami told me her grandmother boiled ginger with lime and honey every time the kids were sick.

She said it worked better than anything from the pharmacy. Cleared congestion. Calmed nausea. Eased sore throats.

I tested it myself when the flu hit me, and I immediately understood why generations have passed it down.

A friend of mine keeps ginger slices in honey for his kids' upset stomachs. One spoonful calms them every time.

Traditional uses: Used across the world for nausea, digestive issues, inflammation, pain, colds, and circulation.

What the research says: Ginger is well-studied. Research shows its effective for nausea (including morning sickness and chemotherapy-induced nausea), can reduce inflammation and muscle pain, and has antimicrobial properties.

How I use it: Fresh root grated into hot water for tea. Added to food. Sliced and stored in honey. Dried and powdered.

Growing ginger in Florida:

Zones: 8-11

Planting: Plant rhizomes in spring, 2-3 inches deep, 8-12 inches apart. Partial shade.

Soil: Rich, well-draining soil. Heavy feeder.

Growth: Grows into tall, leafy plants (2-4 feet) throughout spring and summer.

Harvesting: Dig up rhizomes in fall/winter after leaves die back (8-10 months after planting).

You can harvest small pieces earlier by carefully digging at the edge of the plant without disturbing the whole thing.

Storage: Store fresh in the fridge or freeze. Slice and dry for long-term storage.

Pests: pest-free.

Water: Keep consistently moist during the growing season.

Beginner tip: Fresh ginger is incredibly expensive at the store. Growing your own is a huge money-saver, and the flavor is incomparable.

Safety and precautions:

- Safe in food amounts
- May increase bleeding risk at high doses
- May lower blood sugar
- Can cause heartburn or digestive upset in some people
- If on blood thinners, check with your doctor
- Safe in moderate amounts during pregnancy (often recommended for morning sickness)
- Start with small amounts and increase gradually

Cerasee (Bitter Melon Vine)

Scientific name: Momordica charantia

Cerasee is one of those herbs that carries a story in every Caribbean household.

A woman from Jamaica told me that as a child, she hated it more than anything. Whenever she caught a cold or her stomach was upset, her grandmother would march out to the yard, snip bitter vines, and boil them into deep green tea.

She said the taste was so strong it curled her tongue. But somehow, by the next day, she was always better.

Later in life, when she became a mother, she did the same thing. Brewing that same bitter tea for her own children, passing down the ritual she once dreaded.

That's the story of cerasee. It may taste harsh, but people keep it close because they've seen what it does.

Traditional uses: Used throughout the Caribbean for blood sugar support, digestive issues, skin conditions, and as a general "blood cleanser."

What the research says: Research on bitter melon (the fruit) shows potential benefits for blood sugar management. However, most evidence focuses on the fruit extract, not the leaf tea. The leaves contain similar bioactive compounds, but in different concentrations.

How it's used: Young leaves and stems as tea. People can also eat the ripe fruit (very bitter).

Growing cerasee in Florida:

Zones: 9-11

Planting: Full sun. Give it a trellis or a fence to climb. It's a vigorous vine.

Soil: Tolerates poor soil. Prefers well-draining soil .

Growth: Fast-growing annual vine. Will reseed itself.

Harvesting: Pick young leaves and tender stems. The fruit turns orange when ripe and splits open to reveal red seeds.

Pests: pest-free.

Water: Moderate.

Beginner tip: This vine can take over if you let it. Keep it pruned or contained to one area.

Safety and precautions:

- Very bitter taste; start with weak tea

- May lower blood sugar significantly; monitor closely if diabetic

- Avoid during pregnancy (can stimulate uterine contractions)

- Large amounts may cause digestive upset

- If on diabetes medication, work with your doctor to monitor blood sugar

Although turmeric is part of the Essential Five, combining fresh turmeric and ginger from your yard produces a potent anti-inflammatory tea.

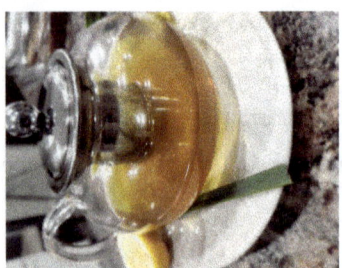

Turmeric, Ginger, and Lemongrass Tea

Building Your Medicinal Garden: Florida-Specific Tips

Location and Layout

Think about placement strategically.

Put taller medicinal trees (soursop, moringa) on the warmest, most protected side of your yard. These create microclimates for more tender plants.

Along sunny edges, plant heat-lovers like lemongrass and ashwagandha.

In partial shade under trees, tuck ginger, turmeric, and shade-tolerant herbs.

In corners or areas you don't visit as often, plant vigorous spreaders like anamu or cerasee.

Use ground covers like sweet potato or perennial peanut between medicinal plants to hold moisture and suppress weeds.

Soil Preparation

Most medicinal herbs prefer well-draining soil rich in organic matter.

In Florida's sand, this means:

- Adding compost liberally
- Mulching heavily (3-4 inches)
- Avoiding tilling (it burns up organic matter in our heat)
- Building soil over time with cover crops and chop-and-drop

For heavy feeders like turmeric and ginger, add extra compost and organic fertilizer.

For drought-tolerant plants like aloe, moringa, and ashwagandha, make sure the drainage is excellent.

Watering

In the dry season (November-April): Water consistently, but not obsessively. Deep watering 2-3 times per week is better than daily shallow watering.

In the wet season (May-October): Many medicinal herbs can handle Florida's rain. Watch for standing water and improve drainage if needed.

Harvesting

Harvest in the morning after the dew dries but before the heat of the day. This is when essential oils and active compounds are at their peak.

Leaves: Pick young, healthy leaves. Avoid damaged or diseased leaves.

Roots: Harvest after the plant has had a full growing season (8-10 months). Wash thoroughly.

Flowers: Pick just as they open fully.

Drying and Storing

Leaves and flowers: Dry slowly in the shade, not in direct sun. Spread on screens or hang in bundles. Good airflow prevents mold.

Once completely dry (leaves should crumble easily), store in glass jars in a cool, dark place.

Roots: Wash thoroughly. Slice thinly for faster drying. Dry in a dehydrator or low oven (under 115°F to preserve compounds). Store whole or grind into powder.

Shelf life: Properly dried and stored herbs last 6-12 months. After that, potency decreases.

Making Tea: The Basics

For leaves and flowers:

- Use 1-2 teaspoons of dried herb per cup of water
- Pour boiling water over the herbs
- Steep covered for 10-15 minutes
- Strain and drink

For roots and bark:

- Use 1 teaspoon dried root per cup of water
- Simmer gently for 20-30 minutes
- Strain and drink

Combinations: Many herbs work better together. Lemongrass + ginger. Turmeric + black pepper. Moringa + cinnamon.

Sweetening: Honey is traditional and adds its own medicinal properties. Add after the tea cools slightly to preserve the honey's enzymes.

Frequency: Start with one cup per day. Observe how your body responds. You can drink some teas, like moringa and lemongrass, daily. Others are better used occasionally or during specific times (cerasee, anamu).

General Safety Guidelines

Start small: Even if an herb is safe, your body might react differently. Start with weak tea and small amounts.

One at a time: When trying a new herb, use it alone first so you can observe effects. Don't combine multiple new herbs.

Listen to your body: If something doesn't feel right, stop using it. Trust your instincts.

Pregnancy and nursing: Doctors advise against many herbs during pregnancy and breastfeeding. When in doubt, avoid.

Medications: Herbs can interact with medications. Research potential interactions or talk to a pharmacist/doctor.

Chronic conditions: If you have chronic health conditions (diabetes, high blood pressure, autoimmune disease, etc.), work with your healthcare provider.

Quality matters: If you're not growing your own, source herbs from reputable suppliers. Contamination and adulteration are genuine issues.

Dosage: More is not better. Herbs are medicine. Respect dosage guidelines.

Breaks: For some herbs, it's wise to take breaks rather than use continuously for months. This prevents your body from adapting and maintains effectiveness.

God Provides

After my father passed, I spent night after night quietly researching herbs. Looking for peace. For strength. For something to help me keep going.

Then one afternoon, my wife came home holding a little packet. Ashwagandha seeds.

She did not know that was the very plant I'd been studying. No idea I'd spent hours reading about it.

She just felt led.

I planted those seeds with trembling hands. Prayed over them. Watched them grow.

And that season reminded me of a truth I hold close: God always provides.

Praise God.

My healing began in that garden. Not just physical healing, but emotional and spiritual healing too.

The garden became a place where I could grieve and grow at the same time. Where I could work with my hands while my heart processed loss. Where I could see life continuing, seeds sprouting, plants thriving, even when everything else felt heavy.

That's the power of a medicinal garden. It's not just about the herbs you harvest. It's about the process. The connection. The reminder that life goes on, that healing is possible, that God still provides.

Reader Challenge: Start Your Medicine Cabinet This Week

Don't just read this chapter and move on. Do something with it.

Here's your challenge:

Pick two plants from this chapter. One tree or shrub, and one herb or vine.

Don't overthink it. Choose the ones that stir something in you. The ones that fit your space or speak to your spirit, or address something you're dealing with.

Get them in the ground this week. Or into pots if all you have is a balcony or a sunny corner.

Label them with the name and the date you planted them. You'll always remember when the journey began.

Over the next few weeks, visit them every day. Touch the leaves. Notice the growth. Talk to them if you feel led.

Within thirty days, harvest just enough from each plant to brew your first cup of tea grown by your own hands.

Find a quiet place to drink it. Notice the taste. The smell. The way it makes you feel.

Write that down. Not just the flavor, but the energy, the calm, the focus, the peace that comes with it.

Tuck that note into your seed packets or gardening journal.

Years from now, you'll look back at those early scribbles as the beginning of something bigger.

The moment you started building your own living medicine cabinet.

One plant at a time.

One cup at a time.

One step toward freedom, health, and connection with the wisdom that came before us.

Now go plant something that heals.

Chapter 8

TIME & MONEY

Everybody loves the idea of a food forest.

Lush greenery everywhere. Fresh fruit within arm's reach. Backyard medicine is growing like weeds. Kids running through rows of banana plants. Avocados dropping into your hands. Moringa in breakfast smoothies. The whole tropical paradise vision.

That picture is beautiful. It's inspiring. It's why most people start.

But here's what nobody talks about in those Instagram posts and YouTube videos: the reality of building and maintaining one.

Too many people plant without thinking about the cost. The upkeep. The years it takes. Whether they actually have the time to take care of what they're building.

That's how you end up with dead trees in the backyard. Wasted money. Frustration. And a lot of "I'll get back to it next season" that never happens.

I've seen it over and over. People go all-in, spend thousands, plant fifty trees in a weekend, then six months later half of them are dead and they're ready to give up completely.

This chapter is about making sure that doesn't happen to you.

Because a food forest is one of the best investments you can make for your family's future. But only if you build it in a way that actually fits your life.

Let's break down the actual costs, the real timeline, and the actual work involved so you can build something sustainable instead of something that burns you out.

The Three Currencies: Time, Money, and Energy

Most people only think about money when they're planning a garden. How much do the trees cost? What about soil? Mulch? Tools?

But money is only one of three currencies you'll spend building a food forest.

The other two are time and energy. And honestly, those two are usually what kill people's gardens, not money.

Let's look at each one.

Currency 1: **Your Time**

If you work 50 hours a week, have three kids, and think you can maintain a half-acre tropical orchard like a full-time farmer, you're lying to yourself.

I don't say that to be harsh. I say it because I've watched people set themselves up for failure by overestimating how much time they actually have.

You need to match your garden's size to the hours you actually have available, not the hours you wish you had or hope to have someday.

Here's the truth: even a small food forest takes time. Especially in the first few years.

You're watering consistently. Mulching. Weeding. Pruning. Watching for pests. Protecting young plants from Florida's heat, storms, and occasional freezes.

Establishing your system significantly reduces the time commitment. Year three, year four, you're spending way less time maintaining and way more time harvesting.

But getting there requires consistent time investment.

Start small. Seriously.

Five productive trees, well-maintained, will feed your family better than twenty neglected trees will.

Get those five thriving. Learn their needs. Build the habits. Then expand.

Reality check: If you can't water your plants three days in a row without skipping, you need to scale back. Either plant fewer things, install drip irrigation, or adjust your expectations.

Currency 2: **Your** money

Let's talk dollars.

You don't need to blow thousands on rare, exotic plants you saw on Instagram. You don't need the $150 grafted mango variety that some people swear is "the best thing ever."

Start with what grows easily and abundantly in your zone first. Get those producing. Then, if you want to splurge on specialty varieties, go for it.

But build your foundation with proven, productive, affordable plants.

Smart spending priorities:

Cheap wins:

- Cuttings (free to a few dollars)
- Seeds (packets for $2-5)
- Trades with neighbors (free)
- Small plants (under $20)
- Mulch from Chip drop or tree services (free or minimal cost)

Worth spending more:

- Mature fruit trees for faster harvests ($50-150)
- Quality tools that last (good pruners, a sturdy shovel, a hose that doesn't kink)
- Drip irrigation setup (saves time and water long-term)
- Good soil amendments and compost for the first year

Here's what people forget: there are ongoing costs.

It's not just the upfront purchase. You'll need soil amendments. Mulch replenishment. Occasional replacement plants when something dies. Pest control materials. Fertilizer if you're not producing enough compost yet.

Budget for maintenance. Not a lot, but something.

A small food forest might cost $20-40 per month in ongoing supplies. A larger one might be $75-150 per month.

That's still way cheaper than buying organic produce every week. But it's not zero. And people get surprised when they haven't planned for it.

Currency 3: **Your Energy**

This one's the hardest to measure, but it's real.

Gardening takes physical energy. You're bending, lifting, digging, hauling mulch, pruning, and carrying water.

In Florida's heat, that's exhausting.

It also takes mental energy. Remembering to water. Noticing when a plant looks off. Researching solutions to problems. Deciding what to plant, where to plant it, and when to prune.

And it takes emotional energy. Dealing with setbacks. Watching plants die despite your best efforts. Staying motivated when progress feels slow.

If you're already running on empty, physically, mentally, or emotionally, starting a massive garden project might not be the move right now.

Maybe you start with three potted herbs on the porch. Build from there as your energy allows.

There's no shame in starting small. In fact, it's smarter.

The Maintenance Reality Nobody Talks About

Here's the brutal truth: neglect will kill a garden faster than any pest ever will.

Marketers often call food forests "low-maintenance" or "self-sustaining."

But getting to that established point takes work. Actual work. For at least two years.

What you'll be doing in years one and two:

Watering consistently. In Florida's dry season, young trees and annual crops need water 2-3 times per week. In the heat of summer, sometimes more.

Mulching heavily. And replenishing it. Mulch breaks down fast in Florida. You'll add more every few months.

Pruning to shape trees and encourage growth. Young fruit trees need training. Herbs and perennials need cutting back to stay productive.

Fighting weeds. They pop up through the mulch. They compete with your plants. You'll pull or chop them back.

Protecting young plants. This protects them from sunscald. Because of cold snaps. From storms. From pests.

Pest management. Checking plants regularly. Hand-picking caterpillars. Spraying organic solutions when needed.

Amending soil. Adding compost. Adjusting the pH if necessary. Building fertility.

That's a lot. And it adds up.

If you plant more than you can realistically maintain, things die. You get discouraged. You quit.

I've seen it happen so many times.

The people who succeed are the ones who plant within their capacity to maintain. They'd rather have ten healthy, thriving plants than thirty struggling, half-dead ones.

The 80/20 Rule of Food Forests

Here's a principle that will save you a lot of frustration: 80% of your harvest will come from 20% of your plants.

Not every tree produces equally. Some plants are absolute workhorses. Others are finicky, low-yielding, or just not suited to your specific microclimate.

Your job is to identify your producers and make them the stars of your system.

Example: I have a papaya tree that's given me fruit almost every week for two years. I also have a mango tree that's been in the ground for three years and hasn't produced a single fruit yet.

The papaya has earned more space. More attention. More propagation. I've planted three more papayas because I know they perform.

The mango? I'm being patient, but I'm not pouring resources into it the way I am with proven producers.

Don't keep investing time and money into a plant that's been struggling for years just because you "should" have it or because it sounds impressive.

If a guava tree is giving you baskets of fruit every season and requires minimal care, that's your MVP. Treat it like one.

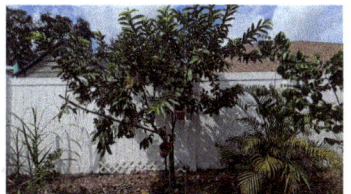
One of my Guava Trees

Systems Save You (and Your Sanity)

If you want this lifestyle to last, you need to set up systems so you're not relying on willpower and memory alone.

Willpower runs out. You get busy. You forget. Life happens.

But systems keep working even when you're tired.

Key systems to implement:

Drip irrigation: Saves time watering. Saves water. Delivers moisture directly to the roots. Set it on a timer and forget about it.

Heavy mulching: Suppresses weeds. Keeps moisture. Moderates soil temperature. Breaks down into compost.

Perennial crops: Plant once, harvest for years. Way less work than replanting annuals every season.

Grouping plants by needs: Put high-water plants together. Put drought-tolerant plants together. Makes watering and care more efficient.

Composting system: Turns waste into soil. Reduces the need to buy amendments. Can be as simple as a pile in the corner.

Chop and drop: Instead of hauling away prunings, chop them up and leave them as mulch where they fall. Feeds the soil. Saves time.

Once your systems are in place, you react less to problems and spend more time harvesting.

The Long Game (And Why Year One Is the Hardest)

A food forest isn't a one-season project. It's a living, long-term investment.

And like any investment, the returns aren't immediate.

Year one: You're spending more than you're getting. You're buying trees, soil, mulch, and tools. You're spending hours setting things up. Your harvest is minimal, mostly from fast growers like herbs, papayas, and bananas.

Year two: You see returns. More plants are producing. Your soil is improving. You're spending less on outside inputs because your compost is ready and your mulch is breaking down into the soil.

Year three: If you've done it right, you're eating and healing from your own land regularly. Your grocery bill has dropped noticeably. The systems are in place. Maintenance time has decreased significantly.

By **year five**, your trees are hitting full production. You have more food than you can eat. You're giving it away. Your yard has become an ecosystem that largely takes care of itself.

The people who win at this are the ones who play the long game and don't quit when year one gets ugly.

Because year one is ugly. Plants die. Money goes out. Time feels wasted. You question whether it's worth it.

But you keep going. And by year three, you look back and realize it was absolutely worth it.

Florida Food Forest: Time, Money, and Reality

Let me give you some real numbers based on my experience and conversations with hundreds of other Florida gardeners.

These are estimates for West Central Florida. Adjust slightly for your specific zone and situation.

Small Food Forest (5-8 fruit trees + herbs and greens)

Initial cost (Year 1): $300-800

- 5-8 small to medium fruit trees: $150-400
- Soil amendments and compost: $50-100
- Mulch: $30-100 (or free from Chip drop)
- Seeds and herb starts: $20-50
- Basic tools if you don't have them: $50-150

Monthly maintenance cost: $20-40

- Mulch replenishment
- Organic fertilizers
- Pest control materials
- Occasional replacement plants

Weekly time commitment: 1-2 hours

- Watering (if no irrigation system)
- Quick weeding and mulching
- Harvest and basic observations

Year 1 harvest expectation: Small but meaningful harvests from fast growers (papayas, bananas, herbs, some greens). Fruit trees won't produce yet unless you bought mature trees.

Medium Food Forest (10-20 fruit trees, mixed crops, diverse understory)

Initial cost (Year 1): $800-2,500

- 10-20 fruit trees: $400-1,200
- Soil amendments: $100-200
- Mulch: $100-300
- Herb and vegetable starts: $50-150
- Seeds: $30-75
- Irrigation setup (optional but recommended): $100-400

- Tools: $100-200

Monthly maintenance cost: $30-75

Weekly time commitment: 3-5 hours

Year 1 harvest expectation: Moderate harvest. Perennials are producing. Early fruit from quicker varieties like papaya, mulberry, and loquat.

Large Food Forest (20-40+ fruit trees, diverse understory, full system)

Initial cost (Year 1): $2,500-6,000+

- 20-40+ fruit trees: $1,000-3,000
- Soil amendments and compost: $300-600
- Mulch: $200-500
- Understory plants: $200-500
- Irrigation system: $300-800
- Quality tools: $200-400
- Seeds and starts: $100-200

Monthly maintenance cost: $75-150+

Weekly time commitment: 6-10 hours

Year 1 harvest expectation: Heavy harvests from quick crops (herbs, greens, sweet potatoes, papayas). First fruit appearing on faster trees. Slower trees like mango and avocado are still establishing.

Full Property Food Forest (½ acre or more, planned system)

Initial cost (Year 1): $6,000-15,000+

This includes professional design consultation, bulk tree purchases, significant irrigation infrastructure, soil amendments at scale, mulch delivery, quality tools, and potentially hiring help for installation.

Monthly maintenance cost: $150-400+

Weekly time commitment: 10-20+ hours (or hire help)

Year 1 harvest expectation: Significant harvest potential from fast growers, but year one is still primarily an establishing phase. The investment pays off in years 2 through 5.

How to Read These Numbers

These estimates assume you're doing the work yourself. Hiring help increases costs significantly, but saves time.

You can reduce initial costs by:
- Starting with small trees or cuttings instead of mature plants
- Sourcing free mulch
- Making your own compost
- Getting plants from neighbors or at plant swaps
- Building your own irrigation system
- Expanding gradually over multiple years instead of all at once

Monthly maintenance costs cover:
- Fertilizer (if not making enough compost yet)
- Mulch replenishment
- Pest management supplies
- Occasional replacement plants
- Seeds for annual crops

Time commitment is actual hands-on work: watering, pruning, harvesting, mulching, pest checks, and planting.

This doesn't include learning time (researching plants, watching videos, reading) or planning time.

The Year 1-3 Commitment Curve

Understanding this curve is critical.

Year 1: Highest time and money investment. Lowest harvest return. This is the hardest year. You're putting in way more than you're getting out.

Year 2: Time and money investment decreased. Harvest increases significantly. You felt the momentum shift.

Year 3: Time and money investment plateau at a low, sustainable level. Harvest increases dramatically. This is when it feels easy and abundant.

Most people quit in year one because they don't understand this curve.

They expect immediate returns. When they don't see them, they assume it's not working.

But it is working. It's just working on nature's timeline, not ours.

Quick Takeaways to Save Time and Money

The bigger you go, the more you need systems. If you're watering by hand past the medium stage, you'll burn out. Install drip irrigation.

Money leaks happen in maintenance. Replacing trees you neglected, buying mulch because you didn't plan for it, treating pests you could have prevented. These costs add up.

Time kills more gardens than pests do. People dream big, plant big, and then can't keep up. Start smaller than you think you need to.

Established food forests are low-maintenance. Getting there is not. Be honest about the work required in years 1-2.

Practical Money-Saving Tips

1. **Buy Smart** with **Fruit Trees**

Check Facebook Marketplace first. Backyard growers in your area often sell trees for cheap, $10-30, surprising you compared to a nursery's $50-100.

Best part? You might only have to drive a few blocks to pick them up.

When buying grafted trees, ask questions. Who grafted it? Who labeled it? How do they know it's the right variety?

Mislabeling happens more than you think.

I once bought what I was told was a 'Lemon Zest' mango tree. Waited three years for fruit. When it finally produced, it was good, but it was definitely not Lemon Zest.

Don't make the same mistake. Ask questions. Buy from reputable sources.

If you're shopping for multiple trees, buy them all on the same day. You can often negotiate bulk discounts. And if you need to rent a truck, it saves money and makes the trip more practical.

Other good places to look:

- Farmer's markets
- Local nurseries (support small businesses, build relationships)
- Your own neighbors (one of mine has a full food forest and sells grafted plants from her yard for next to nothing)

Plant people love to share. Don't be afraid to ask. Half the time they'll give you something for free just because you showed interest.

2. **Don't** stress about buying soil **and** compost **at the** start

You'll see people online bragging about how they make all their own compost and buy nothing from the store.

That's great for them. But nobody starts that way.

We all begin by buying what we need.

Over time, your system will provide mulch, compost, and fertility for itself through chop-and-drop, composting, and natural soil building.

But in the beginning? Buy bagged compost or organic fertilizer from the big-box store if you need to.

It's okay. You're not failing. You're investing in getting your system started.

As your food forest matures, you'll need less from outside sources. But even then, most backyard growers still buy something here and there.

That's normal.

3. Mulch Is Your Best Friend (And It Can Be Free)

Sign up for Chip drop online and you can get wood chips delivered for free.

Here's how it works: arborists need to dump their chips somewhere. You volunteer your property. When a job is nearby, they might drop a load.

The catch? It sometimes works well, and sometimes it doesn't. I waited four years for my first delivery. Others in different areas got theirs in weeks.

Some people tip ($20-50) to encourage faster delivery. It helps.

You can also flag down tree service trucks if you see them hauling away fresh-cut wood in your neighborhood. Slip the crew $20-30 and ask if they'll drop the load at your house instead of driving to the dump.

Nine times out of ten, they'll do it. They'd rather dump it close than drive across town.

Caution: Some people report finding snakes or termites in their chip drop piles. Personally, I've had two drops with no issues. Let the pile sit for a few days before spreading it, and check it first.

4. Start with Productive, Proven Plants

Your first trees should be the ones that produce quickly and reliably in Florida:

Fast producers (harvest in 1-2 years):

- Papaya
- Banana
- Mulberry
- Loquat

- Moringa
- Katuk
- Sweet potatoes

Slower but worth it (harvest in 3-5 years):

- Mango
- Avocado
- Citrus
- Guava
- Longan

Get the fast producers in first so you're getting harvests while waiting for the slower trees to mature.

This keeps you motivated. Keeps you invested. Keeps you from giving up.

The Truth About Gardening as an Investment

Gardening is an investment upfront. It costs money. It takes time. Sometimes it feels like more is going out than coming back.

But give it a few years, and the balance shifts.

Your system produces. Your yard provides. The outside costs shrink.

By year three, the money you're saving on groceries exceeds what you're spending on maintenance.

By year five, it's not even close. You're producing hundreds, sometimes thousands of dollars worth of food annually.

And that's just the financial return.

You're also getting:

- Better health from fresh, chemical-free food
- Physical activity that keeps you strong
- Time outdoors that's good for your mental health

- Skills that last a lifetime
- Something to pass down to your kids
- Food security and independence

You can't put a dollar amount on those things.

But they're real. And they're worth it.

Be patient. Stick with it. You'll see it pay you back many times over.

Make it make sense to you

Here's the last word: make it make sense for your life.

The amount allocated to your budget. Your daily plan. Your climate. The goals you have. Your energy level.

Don't copy what you see online without adapting it to your reality.

Don't build someone else's dream food forest. Build yours.

If you work full time and have young kids, maybe you start with five trees and a handful of herbs. That's enough.

If you're retired with time and energy, maybe you'll go bigger.

If you're on a tight budget, maybe you start with cuttings and seeds and expand slowly over the years.

If you have money to invest upfront, maybe you buy mature trees and irrigation and get producing faster.

There's no right or wrong size. There's only what you can actually maintain.

Because a smaller, well-kept garden will beat a neglected jungle every single time.

A backyard with five thriving mango trees, a patch of sweet potatoes, and a few productive herbs will feed you better than a half-acre of dead and dying plants will.

Start where you are. Build what you can maintain. Expand as your capacity grows.

That's how you create something that lasts. Something that actually works. Something that feeds your family for decades instead of burning you out in six months.

Think long term. Build systems. Be realistic about your time and money.

And remember: you're not just planting trees. You're building a legacy.

Make it one you can sustain.

Chapter 9

WHY I TRAIN LIKE I GROW

The garden saved me once.

But it couldn't save me a second time.

Not alone, anyway.

Let me explain.

When my father passed away , something in me broke I didn't know could break.

The first few weeks after his death, I couldn't look at a weight. Couldn't even think about training. The idea of walking into a gym or doing a workout felt impossible, like trying to speak a language I'd forgotten.

Food became my comfort. Pizza. Fast food. Whatever was easy and made me feel something other than the hollow ache in my chest.

But the decline started months before he died.

During those long hospital visits, watching him fade day by day, I stopped training altogether. Stopped caring about my body. Stopped caring about much of anything except being there with him or talking to him any chance that I could.

The weight crept on. Ten pounds. Twenty. Then more. I stopped looking in mirrors.

After his funeral, after the service, after everyone went home and the house got quiet again, I thought the garden would fix me like it had before.

I'd go outside. Pull weeds. Water trees. Prune branches. And it helped. It did. The garden gave me a place to grieve without words. A place to put my hands on something alive when everything felt dead.

But the weight didn't come off. The heaviness in my chest didn't lift. And every time I caught my reflection, I saw someone I didn't recognize.

I was drowning. And I knew it.

The garden could hold my grief. But it couldn't pull me out of the spiral I was in.

That's when I realized something: your body is part of the garden too.

You can cultivate the most beautiful food forest in the world, but if your body breaks down, weakens, and falls ill, what purpose does it serve?

Harvesting fruit is impossible if your back screams when you bend over. Lifting your arms above your head is necessary for pruning trees. You cannot enjoy the life you are building if you are too tired, too heavy, or too broken to live it.

The garden feeds you. But your body has to be strong enough to work it, enjoy it, and pass it on.

I needed something hard. Something that would force me back into my body. Something that hurt enough to match the pain I was already carrying.

That's when I did the Murph. Every day. For thirty days straight.

What is the Murph?

The Murph workout honors Lieutenant Michael Murphy. Lieutenant Michael Murphy was a Navy SEAL who died in action in Afghanistan in 2005.

Before he died, "Murph" was one of his favorite workouts. It's simple in concept, but absolutely punishing in execution.

Here's what it is:

- 1-mile run
- 100 pull-ups
- 200 push-ups
- 300 air squats
- 1-mile run

All while wearing a 20-pound weight vest if you want to do it the way he did.

Most people do this workout once a year on Memorial Day to honor fallen soldiers and specifically to honor Lieutenant Murphy's sacrifice.

It takes most people 45 minutes to an hour to complete. Some take longer. Elite athletes might finish in under 40 minutes.

It's hard. It's supposed to be hard.

And I did it every single day for thirty days.

People thought I was crazy. My wife looked at me as if I'd lost my mind. And honestly, maybe I had.

But I needed something that would break me down and force me to rebuild. Something that demanded everything I had. Something I couldn't quit halfway through.

I needed to prove to myself that I could still do hard things. That I wasn't just the broken man staring back at me in the mirror.

The First Day (And Why I Almost Quit)

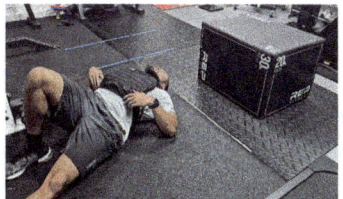
Day One of Murph - In Pain!

Day one was hell.

I could barely finish. My lungs felt as if they were on fire. My arms shook. I felt as though my legs were concrete.

The pull-ups were the worst. I had to break them into sets of five, sometimes three, just to get through a hundred. My hands tore open. Blood mixed with sweat on the bar.

The push-ups weren't much better. My chest screamed. My shoulders gave out. I collapsed face-first into the grass more times than I can count.

The squats? By rep 200, my legs were cramping so badly I thought I might not stand up.

And then I still had to run another mile.

I finished in just over an hour. Collapsed on the ground. Laid there staring at the sky, gasping for air, wondering what I'd just done to myself.

Every part of me wanted to quit. To say, "I tried, it's too hard, I'm done."

But something in me whispered: *Do it again tomorrow.*

So I did.

Day Two Through Thirty: The Shift

The second day was just as hard as the first. My body's previous exhaustion might have made the second day harder.

But I showed up. I documented it. I filmed myself struggling through those pull-ups, grinding through those push-ups, running on legs that didn't want to move.

I posted every single workout on my YouTube channel, @GrowFitFL. Not because I thought people would care. But because making it public meant I couldn't quit quietly.

If I stopped, people would know. And that accountability kept me going on the days when I had nothing left.

Around day seven, something shifted.

The pull-ups got a little easier. Difficult. But easier. I could do sets of ten instead of five.

The push-ups stopped feeling impossible. I could knock out twenty, thirty at a time before needing a break.

The squat became meditative. Just me, my breath, and the count.

By day fifteen, I wasn't just surviving the workout. I was attacking it.

And somewhere in the middle of all that pain, all that sweat, all that struggle, I found something I thought I'd lost.

Myself.

The thing about doing something this hard is that it doesn't leave room for excuses. Negotiations with the Murph are impossible. You can't do half of it and call it good. You can't skip the parts that suck.

You either do it or you don't.

And every day I did it, I was choosing myself. Choosing to fight. Choosing to rebuild what grief had torn down.

The garden gave me peace. But the Murph gave me strength.

By day thirty, I was a different person.

Not just physically, though I'd lost the weight and built muscle I hadn't seen in years.

But mentally. Emotionally. Spiritually.

I'd proven to myself that I could still do hard things. This showed I hadn't sustained irreparable damage. That my father's death didn't have to be the end of my strength.

It could be the beginning of something else. Something forged in fire.

Why Fitness Matters as Much as Food?

Here's what I learned through that experience: you can't separate your body from the rest of your life.

Your physical strength affects everything.

It affects your mental health. Exercise is one of the most powerful tools we have for managing stress, anxiety, and depression. It's not a cure-all, but it's real. The research backs this up over and over.

It affects your longevity. Strength training, in particular, is one of the best predictors of healthy aging. People who maintain muscle mass and strength as they age live longer, healthier lives. They stay independent. They don't end up in nursing homes because they can't get out of a chair.

It affects your food forest. If your back hurts, you can't bend over to harvest sweet potatoes. If your grip is weak, you can't prune branches or carry buckets of mulch. Incapacity in your legs prevents you from walking your property, planting trees, or working the land.

Your garden needs you strong.

It affects your family. Your kids are watching. Their observation focuses on whether you move your body or shy away. They'll see whether you make excuses or show up. They learn what "health" looks like by watching you live it.

It affects your legacy. You're not just building a food forest for yourself. You're building it for your kids, your grandkids, maybe even their kids. But you have to be alive and healthy enough to teach them how to use it.

Fitness is not vanity. It's survival. It's stewardship of the one body you'll ever have.

You can't grow food and ignore your body

I see it all the time. People obsessed with growing the perfect organic tomato while their own body is falling apart.

They'll research soil pH for hours but won't do a single push-up.

They'll spend money on heirloom seeds but won't invest in their own strength.

They'll talk about "natural living" while ignoring the most natural thing humans have done for thousands of years: move heavy things, run, climb, lift, carry.

Here's the truth: if you're growing food but not training your body, you're only doing half the work.

You're feeding yourself from the outside but starving yourself from the inside.

Your muscles need to be fed too. In motion. With resistance. With challenge.

Your cardiovascular system needs to be fed. With running, walking, swimming, anything that makes your heart work.

Your joints and tendons need to be fed. With full range-of-motion movement, stretching, and mobility work.

Your mind needs to be fed. With the endorphins, clarity, and confidence that come from pushing your body past what you thought it could do.

The garden is half of the equation. Your body is the other half.

You Need Both

I need the garden. Staying sane is what this does for me. It feeds my family. It gives me purpose and peace.

But I also need the gym. I need the pull-up bar. I need the weights, the runs, the workouts that make me sweat and struggle.

Because the garden alone couldn't pull me out of the grief spiral I was in after my dad died.

It held me. It gave me a place to be. But it couldn't rebuild the strength I'd lost.

The Murph did that. Thirty days of hell that forced me to confront my weaknesses and do something about it.

And now, years later, I still train. Not thirty days of Murph; that was a onetime thing I needed to break through. But I train consistently. The gym is where I go. I run. I move my body with intention.

Because I know what happens when I don't. I've lived it.

And I'm never going back there.

Your Turn: Why You Need to Move

I know what you're thinking.

Jermaine, fitness isn't my thing.

I've heard every excuse. And trust me, I've used most of them myself.

But here's the thing: you don't have to be a fitness person to move your body.

It's not mandatory to love the gym. You don't have to run marathons. You don't have to do the Murph or anything close to it.

You just have to do something.

Because your body moves. It's designed to lift, carry, push, pull, squat, and run.

And when you stop doing those things, your body breaks down. Your joints become stiff, muscles atrophy, heart weakens. Your bones become fragile.

It's not a matter of if. It's a matter of when.

But the good news is? You can reverse it. At any age. At any fitness level.

You just have to start.

Start Where You Are (Not Where You Think You Should Be)

Let me be very clear: I'm not telling you to go do the Murph.

That was my thing. My battle. My way through grief.

Your starting point is unique. And that's okay.

Maybe your starting point is a ten-minute walk around the block.

Maybe it's five push-ups against the kitchen counter.

Maybe it's three air squats before you sit down to eat.

Maybe it's just standing up from a chair without using your hands.

Start there. Wherever "there" is for you.

The goal isn't to be perfect. The goal is to move.

Build the habit first, worry about the details later

Don't overcomplicate this.

A gym membership is unnecessary. You don't need fancy equipment. You don't need a personal trainer or a perfect program.

You need to move your body consistently.

That's it.

Here's a simple framework that works for anyone, anywhere:

1. **Pick a time**

Same time every day, if possible. Morning works best for most people because life gets in the way later. But whenever works for you, lock it in.

2. **Pick a space**

Your backyard. Your living room. A corner of the bedroom. The porch. Doesn't matter. Just claim a space where you're going to move.

3. Pick a movement

Walking. Push-ups. Squats. Jumping jacks. Pull-ups if you have a bar. Lifting weights if you have . Anything that challenges your body.

4. Do it for ten minutes

That's all. Ten minutes. Every single day.

If you can do more, great. But ten minutes is the non-negotiable minimum.

5. Track it

Write it down. Mark a calendar. Post it on social media if that helps you stay accountable.

The act of tracking makes it real. It builds momentum. It shows you progress when you can't feel it yet.

What if you hate exercise?

Then you haven't found the right movement yet.

Some people hate running but love lifting weights.

Some people hate gyms but love hiking or biking.

Some people hate structured workouts but love playing sports or dancing.

Movement doesn't have to look like a gym bro's Instagram feed. It just has to get your heart rate up and challenge your muscles.

Experiment. Try different things. Find what doesn't make you want to quit after five minutes.

For me, it's a mix. I lift weights because I love feeling strong. Running helps me clear my head. I do bodyweight workouts because they're simple and I can do them anywhere.

You'll find your thing. Just keep trying until you succeed.

What if I'm "too old," or "too out of shape?"

You're not.

I've seen seventy-year-olds build more strength in six months than they had in their fifties.

I've seen people who couldn't walk up a flight of stairs without gasping run 5Ks.

I've seen people who'd been sedentary for decades completely transform their bodies and their lives.

Your body wants to be strong. It's designed for it. You just have to give it the stimulus.

Start where you are. Not where you were twenty years ago. Not where you think you should be. Where you actually are right now.

And build from there. One workout at a time. One day at a time.

Progress isn't linear. Some days will feel great. Some days will feel terrible. That's normal.

What matters is showing up consistently, even on the terrible days.

The Role of Strength in a Food Forest

Let's bring this back to the garden.

Building and maintaining a food forest is physical work.

You're digging holes. Hauling mulch. Carrying buckets of compost. Lifting bags of soil. Pruning branches overhead. Bending over to harvest low-growing crops.

If your body isn't strong, that work becomes painful. Dangerous, even.

I've seen people throw out their backs trying to move a heavy pot. Strain their shoulders reaching for fruit. Hurt their knees squatting to pull weeds.

Not because they're doing it wrong. Their bodies are unprepared for the work.

Strength training prepares you for real life.

Squats make it easier to get up and down from the ground.

Deadlifts teach you how to lift heavy things safely.

Pull-ups build the back and grip strength you need for pruning and carrying.

Push-ups strengthen your chest and shoulders for lifting bags and moving wheelbarrows.

Core work stabilizes your spine so you don't hurt yourself bending and twisting.

When you train your body intentionally, the work in the garden becomes easier. Your movement is less painful. You recover faster. You can work longer without breaking down.

And that means you can actually enjoy the garden instead of just surviving it.

Your home gym doesn't have to be fancy

You don't need a garage full of equipment to get strong.

Here's what I recommend for a simple, effective home gym that covers everything you need:

A pull-up bar ($20-50): Installs in a doorway. Builds back, arms, and grip strength. One of the best investments you can make.

Resistance bands ($15-30): Versatile, portable, effective. You can do hundreds of exercises with a set of bands.

A pair of dumbbells ($30-100 depending on weight): Start with whatever weight challenges you for 8-12 reps. You can do a full-body workout with just two dumbbells.

A yoga mat ($15-30): For floor exercises, stretching, and core work.

That's it. Less than $200 total, and you have a complete home gym.

If you want to expand later, add a kettlebell, a jump rope, or a weight vest.

But those four things (pull-up bar, bands, dumbbells, mat) will get you incredibly strong if you use them consistently.

The beauty of a home gym is that it removes excuses.

Avoid driving across town. There is no waiting for equipment. No monthly fees. Not feeling self-conscious in front of other people.

You walk into your garage, your spare room, or even just your backyard, and you train.

Simple. Effective. Sustainable.

A Simple Workout to Start With

If you don't know where to start, here's a simple full-body workout you can do with minimal equipment:

Warm-up (5 minutes):

- Arm circles
- Leg swings
- Jumping jacks or high knees
- Bodyweight squats

Workout (20-30 minutes):

- Push-ups: 3 sets of as many as you can do (change on knees if needed)
- Squats: 3 sets of 15-20 reps
- Rows (with bands or dumbbells): 3 sets of 10-12 reps
- Plank: 3 sets of 30-60 seconds
- Lunges: 3 sets of 10 per leg

Cool-down (5 minutes):

- Stretching (hamstrings, quads, chest, shoulders)
- Deep breathing

Do this three times a week. Monday, Wednesday, Friday. Or Tuesday, Thursday, Saturday. Whatever fits your schedule.

On the other days, walk. Move. Stay active. But give your muscles time to recover.

As you get stronger, add weight. Add reps. Add sets. Make it harder.

But start simple. Master the basics. Build the habit.

The Mental and Emotional Benefits You Don't Expect

Here's what nobody tells you about exercise: the physical benefits are only half the story.

The mental and emotional benefits are just as powerful, maybe more so

Exercise reduces anxiety and depression. It's as effective as medication for mild-to-moderate cases, and it has zero negative side effects.

Exercise improves sleep. You fall asleep faster, sleep deeper, and wake up feeling more rested.

Exercise boosts confidence. Every time you complete a workout, you prove to yourself that you can do hard things. That confidence spills into every other area of your life.

Exercise clears your mind. There's something about moving your body that quiets the mental noise. You come out of a workout with more clarity than you went in with.

Exercise gives you control. In a world where so much is outside your control, your body is something you can work on, improve, and take ownership of.

After my dad died, I felt powerless. Like everything was falling apart and I couldn't stop it.

But when I did the Murph, I had control. I have completed it. Every day, I made an appearance. I finished every rep.

And that control, that small daily victory, gave me back a sense of agency I desperately needed.

Exercise can do that for you too.

The Garden and the Gym: Two Sides of the Same Coin

Your health is not one thing. It's a system.

What you eat matters. What you grow matters. Your movement makes a difference. How you think matters. How you rest matters.

The garden feeds you from the outside in.

The gym builds you from the inside out.

Together, they create a foundation for a strong, healthy, long life.

You can't have one without the other and expect to thrive.

I've seen people who eat perfectly but never move. They're thin but fragile, prone to injury.

I've seen people who train hard but eat garbage. They're strong but inflamed, sick, running on borrowed time.

The people who thrive? They do both.

They grow actual food and eat it. They move their bodies and make them strong.

That's the goal. Not perfection. Balance.

Your Challenge: Thirty Days of Something

I will not tell you to do the Murph for thirty days. That was my journey, not yours.

But I am going to challenge you to do something for thirty days.

Pick one movement. One workout. One physical challenge.

It could be:

- A daily walk (even just ten minutes)
- Ten push-ups every morning
- A plank hold (start with 20 seconds, build up)
- Five pull-ups (or work toward your first one)
- A simple bodyweight circuit three times a week

Whatever it is, commit to it for thirty days.

Track it. Write it down. Post it online if that helps you stay accountable.

And on day thirty, notice how you feel.

Not just physically. Mentally. Emotionally.

Notice your energy. The way you are feeling. Your confidence. Your clarity.

I promise you, something will shift.

It won't be dramatic.

But by day thirty, you'll feel different. Stronger. More capable. More alive.

And that feeling will make you want to keep going.

Final Thoughts: You Can't Pour from an Empty Cup

You're building a food forest to take care of your family. To give them actual food, health, security, and independence.

That's beautiful. That's worth doing.

But you can't take care of them if you're not taking care of yourself.

You can't pour from an empty cup.

Your broken, weak, and sick body prevents you from doing the work. You can't enjoy the harvest. You can't pass on the knowledge.

Your body is part of the garden. Treat it like one.

Feed it. Train it. Rest it. Care for it.

Not because you want to look a certain way or impress anyone.

But because you have work to do. People who need you. A legacy to build.

And you need to be strong enough to see it through.

So plant your trees. Grow your food. Build your systems.

But don't forget to build yourself too.

Your family needs a garden. But they need you even more.

Make sure you're strong enough to give them both.

Chapter 10

THE HOME TRILOGY

If I could only pass down three things to my children, it wouldn't be money.

It wouldn't be property or possessions or anything you could sell.

It would be three practices. Three pillars. Three disciplines that have saved my life more times than I can count.

It's a garden. This is a gym. That is a library.

Their impressive appearance is not the reason. Not because they make good content for social media. Not because anyone else says they matter.

But because they're the three tools that keep me alive, sharp, and moving forward no matter what the world is doing.

These three things, built into your home and woven into your life, will carry you through anything. Loss. Chaos. Economic collapse. Personal crisis. Grief that feels like it will swallow you whole.

I know because they've carried me.

Let me show you why.

The Garden: Food is Freedom

In the world right now, depending on the grocery store for everything you eat is a gamble you're taking, whether you realize it.

Prices jump overnight. Quality drops. Shelves empty when systems break. And you have zero control over what people spray on your food, how it grows, or how long it sits in a truck, slowly losing nutrients.

That's not security. That's dependency.

When I walk into my backyard, I see something different.

Mango trees heavy with fruit that I planted years ago. Herbs growing thick and green that double as medicine. Sweet potatoes sprawling across beds I built with my own hands. Soil that's alive because I've fed it, tended it, learned it.

That's not just food. That's insurance. It's freedom. It's trust.

I know what went into that soil. I know what's on those leaves. I know I picked the fruit at a specific time.

And when the world gets uncertain, when prices spike or supply chains break or headlines scream about shortages, I don't panic.

Because I have food in the ground.

That's a different wealth. The kind you can't buy at any price once you actually need it.

Key truth: When you control your food, you control your health, your wallet, and your peace of mind.

But here's the deeper part that most people miss.

The garden doesn't just feed your body. It feeds something else, too.

When you plant a seed and watch it grow, you remember something fundamental about how the world works. You remember that life continues. That things grow even when everything else feels like it's falling apart. That you can create, not just consume.

After my father died, the garden held me when nothing else could. It gave me a place to put my grief, my hands, my energy. It gave me something to tend when I couldn't fix anything else.

The garden doesn't judge. It doesn't ask questions. It just grows.

And in watching things grow, you believe you can grow too. That you can compost your broken parts into something fertile. That death isn't the end of the story.

The garden teaches you patience. It teaches you that good things take time. That you can't rush a mango tree or force a tomato to ripen before it's ready.

It teaches you resilience. Because you will fail. Plants will die. Pests will come. Storms will knock things down. And you'll have to get back up, replant, and try again.

It teaches you stewardship. That some things are worth tending even when the payoff is years away. That you can plant trees you'll never fully harvest because the people who come after you will need shade and fruit.

The garden is not just about food. It's about becoming the person who can sustain life. Who can create abundance? Who doesn't wait for someone else to provide?

And once you understand that, you realize the garden is one of the most radical acts of resistance you can commit in a world designed to keep you dependent.

For every tomato you cultivate, you avoid purchasing one. Every herb you harvest is medicine you didn't have to pay for. Every tree you plant is food your children won't have to purchase.

That's freedom.

Not the kind you vote for or protest for, or hope someone gives you.

The kind you build with your own hands, one seed at a time.

The Gym: Strength is Survival

Let me be straight with you.

I'm not training to look good for Instagram. I'm not chasing abs or trying to impress anyone at the beach.

I'm training because I still want to build my garden when I'm seventy.

I'm training because I want to lift fifty pounds of compost without thinking about it. Because I want to climb a ladder to prune a tree without worrying that my knees will give out. Because I want to carry my grandchildren when they're tired and play with them without getting winded.

I'm training because strength is survival.

And survival isn't just about making it through the day. The topic is thriving. It's about being capable. It's about not being a burden.

Strength training isn't vanity. It's maintenance. It's preparing your body for the work of living.

Your body is a tool. And like any tool, if you don't maintain it, it breaks down.

Think about it. If you had a truck you needed to rely on, you'd change the oil, rotate the tires, and keep it running smooth. You wouldn't let it sit unused until the engine seized.

But somehow, we treat our bodies worse than we treat our vehicles.

They could rust by us. We let them weaken. We ignore the warning signs until something breaks, and then we act surprised.

Strength doesn't just happen. And it doesn't last if you don't work for it.

Every year you don't train, you lose muscle. Your bones grow weaker and your balance deteriorates. Your metabolism slows down. You become more likely to sustain an injury.

But here's the good news: you can reverse it. At any age. With consistent work.

I've seen seventy-year-olds build more strength in six months than they had at sixty. I've seen people who couldn't get up from the floor without help learn to do squats, lunges, and push-ups.

Your body wants to be strong. It's designed for it. You just have to give it a reason.

And the reasons are everywhere.

If the world slows down, if systems break, if help doesn't come when you call, will you be able to take care of yourself? Your family? Your property?

Are you capable of lifting heavy objects? Is it possible for you to transport water? Can you work your land? Can you protect what's yours?

Strength is security. It's independence. It's the ability to say, "I can handle this."

But beyond survival, there's something deeper.

Strength changes how you see yourself.

When you do something you thought was impossible, when you lift a weight you couldn't lift last month, when you finish a workout that almost broke you, something shifts inside.

You believe in yourself differently. You trust that you're capable of hard things.

And that confidence bleeds into every other area of your life.

The discipline you build in the gym shows up in your work, your relationships, and your ability to handle stress. The mental toughness you develop pushing through a hard set translates to pushing through hard seasons.

The gym isn't just about building your body. It's building your mind. You will. Your belief that you can overcome.

Key truth: The stronger you are, the more you can do for yourself, your family, and your future.

And here's what people don't talk about: training your body is an act of gratitude.

You have a body that works. That moves. That can get stronger.

Not everyone does.

Some people would give anything to walk, to lift, to run, to do the things you're choosing not to do because it's inconvenient or uncomfortable.

Every time you train, you're honoring the gift of a working body. You're saying, "I will not waste this. I'm going to strengthen it. I'm going to make it last."

That's sacred work.

So when you clear a corner of your garage or your living room, when you set up a pull-up bar or buy a pair of dumbbells, you're not just building a gym.

You're building a place where you become who you need to be. Where you forget the strength to carry what life hands you.

The Library: Wisdom is Leverage

The garden feeds my body. The gym keeps me capable.

But the library? That's where the real leverage comes from.

I'm not talking about shelves of books you never open, bought to look smart or fill space.

I'm talking about a personal archive of knowledge that you actually use. Books you return . Wisdom you can apply. Information that makes you more capable, more informed, and freer.

Gardening guides that teach you how to grow food in your specific climate. Herbal medicine references that show you which plants can heal. Cookbooks that help you turn your harvest into meals. Financial literacy books that teach you how to manage money. History that shows you how people survived hard times before. Biographies of people who did hard things and lived to tell about it.

This is your proper education. Not the one someone else designed for you, but the one you choose for yourself.

The internet is nice. Until it's not.

When the power goes out. Until the information you need gets buried under memberships, algorithms, and noise. Until the platform changes and the article you saved disappears.

A physical library doesn't have that problem.

You own it. You control it. It sits on your shelf waiting for you, no Wi-Fi required, no subscription needed, no terms of service that can change overnight.

Books are the most concentrated form of wisdom that humanity has ever created. Someone spends years, sometimes decades, learning something, then distills it into a few hundred pages you can read in a weekend.

That's leverage.

You can learn from people who are dead, from people on the other side of the world, from people who've lived through things you'll hopefully never face.

You can compress decades of experience into days of reading. You can stand on the shoulders of giants without ever meeting them.

But only if you have the books. Only if you make the library.

Key truth: Knowledge is power, but only if you own it and know how to use it.

Here's what I've learned: the quality of your library determines the quality of your thinking.

If you only consume social media, shallow articles, and headlines, your thinking will be shallow. Reactive. Fragmented.

But if you read deeply, widely, and intentionally, your thinking changes. Patterns become apparent. You connect ideas. You develop frameworks that help you navigate complexity.

You become someone who understands how things work, not just someone who reacts to what's happening.

And in uncertain times, that's the difference between thriving and barely surviving.

Sudden price increases do not faze a person with knowledge of food cultivation. The person who knows how to fix things doesn't panic when supply chains break. The person who's read history doesn't panic when the headlines scream about collapse, because they know humanity has survived worse.

Knowledge creates calm. It creates options. It creates the ability to adapt.

And that's what a library gives you.

Not answers to every question, but the tools to figure things out. The confidence that if you don't know something, you can learn it. The humility to know you don't have to start from scratch because someone has already walked this path.

Start small. One book this month. One book that will still matter in five years.

Don't buy books to impress people. Buy books that will make you more capable.

Publications about skills. Books on systems. Books on how to think, build, grow, heal, adapt.

And then read them. Mark them up. Dog-ear the pages. Return to them when you need them.

A library isn't decoration. It's a tool. Treat it like one.

The Power of the Trilogy

Here's the truth about these three things: you can survive with of them for a while.

But life will be harder. Weaker. More fragile.

Without the garden, you're spending more money and trusting strangers with your health. You depend feeds on systems you don't control. You're one supply chain disruption away from empty shelves.

Without the gym, you're weaker and more vulnerable. Your body breaks down faster. You become dependent on others for things you used to do yourself. You lose the ability to handle physical challenges when they come.

Without the library, you're at the mercy of whatever information someone else feeds you. Verification is not possible. You can't learn independently. You're relying on experts and authorities who may or may not have your best interests at heart.

But together?

Together, they make you dangerous in the best way possible.

Self-sufficient. Healthy. Learning is a continuous process for me. It is always growing. The construction process is ongoing.

You are not awaiting rescue from anyone. You do not seem to hope for improvement. Systems that don't care about you do not have your dependence.

You're creating your own security. Your own health. Your own knowledge base.

And that makes you free.

Not free in some abstract sense. Free in a real, tangible, walk-it-out-every-day sense.

You are free to feed yourself. Free to move your body. You are free to form your own opinions. Free to build a life that doesn't crumble when the world shakes.

That's the power of the trilogy.

Putting It into Practice

You don't need an enormous property, a fancy gym, or a massive library to start.

You need to start. Period.

Garden: Start with a few raised beds or even containers. Grow food you actually eat. Add a medicinal herb or two. Just one mango tree. One moringa. One pot of basil. Just start.

Gym: Clear a corner of your garage or living room. A pair of dumbbells, resistance bands, a pull-up bar, and your own body weight will do more than you think. You don't need a warehouse full of equipment. You need consistency and effort.

Library: Buy one physical book this month that will still be valuable five years from now. Not fluff. Not trends. Something that builds skills, deepens understanding, or teaches you how to create, fix, or grow something. Keep adding to it, one book at a time.

That's it. That's the start.

Small steps. Consistent action. Long-term thinking.

You're not building this overnight. You've been building it over the years.

But every seed you plant, every workout you complete, every book you read, you're moving closer to a life that's truly yours. A life that doesn't depend on fragile systems or broken promises.

A life rooted in something real.

The Fortress You Build

Garden. Gym. Library.

Those three, built into your home, will outlast markets, storms, and whatever the headlines say is falling apart.

The garden feeds your body with food you can trust. Food you can walk outside and touch with your own hands. Food that doesn't come with a barcode or a mystery ingredient list.

The gym gives you strength. Not just to lift weights, but to carry your children when they're tired. To move soil and build things. To shoulder the work that builds a life worth living.

The library sharpens your mind, fills it with wisdom, and keeps your vision steady when the world is spinning in confusion.

Together, they form a fortress.

Not the kind made of concrete and steel, but the kind rooted deep in the soul.

The kind no one can take from you.

Because here's what I know: systems fail. Institutions crumble. Governments change. Markets crash. Supply chains break.

But the food you grow doesn't disappear because a store closes. The strength you build doesn't vanish because a gym shuts down. The knowledge you own doesn't evaporate because a website goes offline.

What you build in your own home, with your own hands, on your own terms, that lasts.

This makes up the work. That's the calling. That's freedom.

And I will keep building these three things for as long as I live.

Because when you have food in the ground, strength in your body, and wisdom in your mind, you are not at the mercy of the world.

You can weather loss. You can stand steady through chaos. With roots deep enough to outlast you, you can raise a family.

The garden keeps you alive. Strength is what the gym provides. The library keeps you free.

That is the trilogy I've built my life on, and it has carried me through grief, storms, and seasons when it felt like the ground itself was giving way.

It will carry you too.

But only if you build it.

So start today. Plant something. Move your body. Read something that matters.

Just one step. Just one seed. One rep. One page.

Build the trilogy.

Build the fortress.

Build a life that no one can take away.

Because in the end, that's all that matters. Your knowledge is more important than your possessions. Not what you buy, but what you build. Not what others give you, but what you create for yourself.

Your garden, home gym, and personal home library.

There are three pillars. Three practices. Three paths to freedom.
This is the way.
Now go build it.

Chapter 11

MENTAL HEALTH

One morning last year, I woke up with my mind already spinning. Deadlines. Bills. Family stuff. World news. All of it piling up before my feet even hit the floor.

I poured some coffee, but it didn't help. The noise in my head just got louder. I knew staying in the house, whether scrolling my phone or staring at my to-do list, would trap me in that headspace all day.

So I grabbed my hat and walked out into the food forest.

The grass was still wet with dew. The air had that heavy Florida humidity that sits on your chest. But the birds were singing as if it were the best morning they'd ever had, completely unbothered by whatever was weighing me down.

I started pulling weeds around the katuk. Trimming back some moringa that had gotten too tall. Checking the passion fruit vines for fresh growth.

My hands moved. My body followed. And somewhere in those movements, something shifted.

Thirty minutes in, I realized my breathing had slowed. My thoughts had cleared. The weight I woke up with wasn't sitting on my chest anymore.

That's when it hit me, again, like it's hit me a hundred times before: the garden doesn't just grow food.

It grows me.

And I don't mean that in some poetic, abstract way. I mean it literally. Measurably. In ways I can feel in my body and see in how I show up for my family.

The garden has saved my mental health more times than I can count. And I'm not the only one.

There's science behind this now. Real research shows what gardeners have known for generations: dirt heals.

Let me show you how.

The Science of Soil and Sanity

Here's something most people don't know: there's a bacterium in soil called Mycobacterium vaccae that actually affects your brain chemistry.

When you breathe it in or it enters through minor cuts on your hands, it triggers the release of serotonin, the same neurotransmitter that antidepressants target.

Literally, putting your hands in the dirt can make you feel better. Not because it's relaxing (though it is), but because the soil itself contains natural antidepressants.

A study published in *Neuroscience* showed that mice exposed to this soil bacterium displayed less anxiety and better stress resilience. When researchers removed the exposure, the benefits lasted for weeks.

We're not mice, obviously. But the principle holds. Contact with soil, with the microbial world we grew alongside, has measurable effects on mood and mental health.

And that's just one piece.

Multiple studies have shown that gardening reduces cortisol, the stress hormone that spikes when you're overwhelmed. One study in the Journal of Health Psychology found that after a stressful task, people who gardened for 30 minutes had significantly lower cortisol levels than people who read indoors.

Another study in *Preventive Medicine Reports* followed people who gardened regularly and found they had better mental well-being, lower stress, and higher life satisfaction than non-gardeners.

And research published in the International Journal of Environmental Research and Public Health showed that even just viewing nature or being in green spaces reduces anxiety, improves mood, and enhances cognitive function.

This is not woo-woo. This is not some hippie talk. Peer-reviewed and documented science is what this is.

Your brain needs nature. Your nervous system needs it. And when you deny yourself that connection, you pay a price.

But when you step outside, put your hands in the soil, and tend something living, your body responds. Your mind calms. Your stress decreases.

I didn't need the studies to tell me this. I've lived it.

But knowing the science helps me understand why it works. And it helps me take it seriously, not as a luxury or a hobby, but as a necessity.

Nature Doesn't Rush (And Neither Should You)

Out here in the garden, nothing moves at social media speed.

A mango tree doesn't care about trending topics. Seeds don't feel FOMO. Nature moves slow and steady, and if you hang around long enough, you'll match that pace.

That's hard for most of us. We live in a world that's constantly speeding up. All is rapid. Everything is urgent. Everything demands your attention right now.

But the garden operates on a different clock.

You cannot rush a seed. You can't force a tree to fruit before it's ready. Making something grow faster is not possible just because of impatience.

All you can do is tend to it. Water it. Give it time.

And in doing that, you learn something critical: not everything needs to happen right now.

Some things take months. Some take years. And that's okay.

When you're forced to slow down, when you have no choice but to wait for nature's timeline, you notice things you'd otherwise miss.

The way the sun strikes the leaves in the morning, illuminating them from behind, is quite something. How bees move from flower to flower with a focus and purpose that puts my scattered attention to shame. How a plant you thought was done, finished, dead, kicks out fresh growth when conditions are right.

Those small observations, those quiet moments, they rewire something in your brain.

You stop needing everything to be fast and immediate. You appreciate the slow unfolding of things.

That's the first gift the garden gives my mental health: permission to slow down without guilt.

And that's huge for me. Because I'm the type that's always moving, always thinking ahead, always grinding toward the next thing.

The garden tells me it's okay to just be. To exist without producing. To enjoy the process instead of rushing to the result.

In a world that constantly tells you-you aren't doing enough, that message is like medicine.

The Power of Presence

In the garden, I'm not replaying yesterday's arguments.

I'm not stressing over next month's bills, nor wondering if I'm doing enough for my kids, nor worrying about what's happening in the world.

I'm focused on right now. This moment. This plant. The branch right here. This leaf.

Pulling weeds. Smelling lemongrass. Checking for pests. Feeling the soil to see if it needs water.

There's something about putting your hands in the dirt, about working with something alive, that shuts down the mental noise.

You're reminded that life isn't all in your head. It's happening right in front of you. In your hands. Under your feet.

People call it mindfulness. Being fully present in the moment instead of lost in thought.

Therapists charge a lot of money to teach people how to do this. Apps and courses promise to help you "find presence."

But the garden gives it to you for free.

You don't have to meditate or chant or sit cross-legged. You just have to show up and work.

And in that work, in the repetition of simple tasks, your mind settles.

That shift, even for 20 minutes, can reset my entire day.

I've had mornings where I woke up with my mind racing, thoughts crashing into each other, anxiety building before I even knew what I was anxious about.

But by the time I'm done watering and pruning, by the time my hands have touched soil and leaves and stems, my breathing has slowed. I can think straight again.

The heaviness lifts.

And I walked back into the house a different person than the one who had walked out.

That's not an exaggeration. That's a pattern I've lived through hundreds of times.

The garden pulls me out of my head and back into my body. And that's where healing happens.

Gardening as Therapy Without the Couch

Therapy comes in many forms.

For some people, it's sitting on a couch talking to a professional. And that's valuable. I'm not dismissing that.

But for me, kneeling in the soil and planting something new has the same effect. It helps me process. It helps me work through things I don't have words for.

Every hole I dig is a chance to put something in the ground that will give back later. That's hope you can touch. Hope you can water it. Hope that grows, whether you believe in it.

I've planted through grief. Through stress. Through moments when I didn't know what was coming next in life.

And without fail, the act of planting makes me feel lighter.

It's a reminder that I can create good things even when life feels heavy. That I can invest in the future even when the present is hard. That growth is still possible even when everything feels stuck.

After my father passed away, I couldn't talk about it for a long time. The words wouldn't come. The grief sat in my chest like a stone.

But I could plant. I could dig. I could water.

And in doing that, something moved. The grief didn't disappear, but it had somewhere to go. The garden held it for me.

On rough days now, harvesting a basket of fruit is my proof: progress is happening. Even if it's slow. Even if I don't notice it day to day.

The plants don't lie. If I've been tending them, they grow. If I've been watering, they produce.

And that's a powerful reminder when your brain is telling you nothing you do matters, when depression whispers that you're not making progress, when anxiety convinces you everything is falling apart.

The garden says otherwise.

Look, there's fruit. There's fresh growth. There's life where you planted death.

You're doing better than you think.

Movement That Heals

When your body moves, your brain changes.

This isn't motivational talk. It's neuroscience.

Physical movement reduces anxiety and depression. This thing makes you feel better. This can clear brain fog. It helps you sleep better. It gives you more energy during the day.

And gardening? Gardening is full-body movement.

Bending, squatting, reaching, lifting, carrying, and walking are all actions you're performing. You're engaging muscles. You're moving in ways that most of us don't anymore because we sit at desks all day.

That movement tells your nervous system: we're okay. We're safe. We're capable. Keep going.

Research backs this up. A meta-analysis in Environmental Health found that people who gardened regularly had significantly lower rates of depression and anxiety compared to non-gardeners.

Another study in the Journal of Psychiatric Research showed that even light gardening activity for 30 minutes three times a week reduced symptoms of depression as much as moderate-intensity exercise.

I didn't need the research to know this. I've lived it.

I've had days where I could feel the tension building in my shoulders, my jaw tight, my mood flat, my patience thin.

A few hours in the yard, moving and sweating, working and breathing, can flip that completely.

The physical work pulls the stress out of me like the soil pulls in water.

And I came back inside calmer. Clearer. More patient with my kids. More present with my wife.

That's not just about feeling better in the moment. That's about being a better man. A better father. A better husband.

The garden makes me someone I'm proud to be.

A Living Reminder That Seasons Change

Every plant in my yard is proof that hard seasons end.

I've seen trees stripped by storms bounce back stronger the next year. I've seen dry patches turn lush after a single rain. I've had plants I gave up on, plants I thought were dead, surprise me months later with fresh shoots.

What looked dead was just waiting for the right time.

That's how life works, too.

When you live with that truth in front of you every day, when you see it with your own eyes in the leaves and branches and fruit, it's harder to believe that a terrible season will last forever.

Because the garden teaches you: this too shall pass.

When the dry season ends, the wet season begins. The cold snaps pass. The heat breaks.

Nothing stays the same. And that's good news when you're in the middle of hard times.

You're not stuck here. This isn't permanent. Things will shift.

Just like the garden.

Just keep tending. Keep showing up. Keep watering even when it feels pointless.

Because the season will change. And when it does, you'll be glad you didn't quit.

The Connection You Can't Buy

When you grow food, you connect to something bigger than yourself.

Your weather predictions are usually accurate. The rainfall patterns are noticeable to you. You observe the phases of the Moon. You pay attention to the soil, the insects, and the birds.

You care about things most people scroll past.

And that connection, that awareness of being part of a larger living system, keeps you grounded in a world that's trying to pull you in a hundred different directions.

You can't buy that kind of grounding. Grow it.

Modern life disconnects you from nature. From your body. From actual work and actual food, and genuine community.

Everything comes through screens. Everything is fast and disposable and shallow.

But when you step into the garden, all of that falls away.

You're connected to the earth beneath your feet. To the sun on your skin. To the plants you're tending with your hands.

That connection is ancient. It's what humans did for thousands of years before we built cities and factories and digital lives.

And your nervous system knows it. Your body recognizes it. Your soul responds to it.

You were made for this. Not sitting in a cubicle under fluorescent lights. Not staring at screens for ten hours a day.

You worked with your hands. To cultivate plants. To be outside. To move your body. To create.

And when you return to that, even for a few hours a week, something in you relaxes.

You remember who you are underneath all the noise.

Practical Ways to Grow Your Mental Health

Let me give you some simple, actionable ways to use the garden for your mental health.

These aren't theories. These are practices that work for me and for hundreds of people I've talked to over the years.

1. **Start your morning outside before screens**

Even ten minutes. Before you check your phone, before you turn on the news, before the world gets its hooks in you, step outside.

Walk your garden. Water something. Just breathe the air.

Let your first input of the day be nature, not chaos.

That sets the tone for everything that follows.

2. **Plant something small and check it daily**

Try a pot of basil. Or maybe a tomato plant. A single herb.

Something that needs your attention.

And every day, check on it. Notice the changes. Water it if it needs it.

Let it be your reminder that progress takes time. That small, consistent actions compound. That growth happens even when you're not watching.

3. **Work with your hands**

Pull weeds. Prune branches. Repot plants. Harvest vegetables.

Let your body lead your mind.

When your hands are busy with simple, repetitive tasks, your mind can process things it doesn't have time for during the busy, loud, distracted hours of the day.

Therefore, people think clearly in the shower or while walking. Your conscious mind's occupation allows your subconscious to work.

Gardening does the same thing.

4. **Make the garden a no-phone zone**

Protect that mental space.

Keep your phone inside. Don't take pictures for social media every time. Don't check texts while you're watering.

Let the garden be a place where you're fully present, fully disconnected from the digital noise.

That boundary is sacred. If you are like me and create content to help others schedule times. Gardening without distractions is one of the many joys of having a garden in the first place; I want you to experience for yourself.

5. **Share your harvest**

Helping others can lift your own mood more than you think.

When you grow more than you need, when you give bags of fruit or vegetables to neighbors, friends, and family, you're not just being generous.

You're connecting, contributing, and now a part of something bigger than yourself.

And that fights isolation, loneliness, and the feeling that what you do doesn't matter.

It matters. The food in that bag proves it.

6. Let yourself fail without judgment

Plants die. That's part of gardening.

You'll over-water something. Underwater something else. Plant in the wrong spot. Choose the wrong variety for your climate.

And that's okay.

The garden doesn't judge you for failing. It just gives you another chance to try.

Let that teach you self-compassion. Let that remind you that failure isn't final; it's feedback.

7. Notice what you're grateful for

Gratitude is one of the most powerful mental health tools we have. And the garden is full of things to be grateful for.

It's the rain that helps your plants grow, aided, of course, by the sun. The soil that holds them. The harvest that feeds you.

Take a moment, even just a few seconds, to notice those things and say thank you.

Not to anyone in particular. Just say it.

That simple practice rewires your brain. It trains you to see abundance instead of scarcity. Blessings instead of problems.

Mental Health Isn't Something You Fix Once

Here's the truth: mental health isn't something you "fix" and then you're done.

It's something you keep tending, like a garden.

Some days are light and days you feel strong. Some days you barely get out of bed.

That's normal. That's human.

But if you keep showing up, if you keep putting your hands in the soil, if you keep watering and planting and tending, you'll see growth.

Within your plants. In your mind. In your life.

The garden grows food. But it also grows patience, gratitude, resilience, and peace.

That's why I say: mental health grows here.

And the best part?

It doesn't matter if you're on an acre, a balcony, or a windowsill.

If you care for a plant, you're also caring for yourself.

You're saying: I deserve to tend something. I deserve to create. I deserve to be connected to life.

And that simple act, repeated over time, can save you.

It saved me.

It can save you too.

So get involved. Plant something. Water it. Watch it grow.

And notice, over time, how you grow with it.

That's the garden's gift. Not just food. Not just beauty.

Healing.

And we all need that.

Chapter 12

RAISING HEALTHY KIDS

I have four children.

Four completely distinct personalities, spread across a huge age gap. My oldest is practically an adult. My youngest is still learning to walk.

My wife and I had our last baby in our 40s, which means we're doing the whole diaper-and-sleepless-nights thing again while also helping the older ones navigate teenage drama and life decisions.

People ask me all the time: "How do you do it? How do you stay healthy with four kids? How do you teach them about food and fitness when the world is working against you?"

And here's my answer: I look around at the world we're raising our kids in, and it's a mix of opportunity and danger.

There's more information available than ever before. We can provide further resources. More technology. More ways to learn and grow.

But there's also more junk in our food. Within our environment. In our media. In our minds.

It scares me sometimes, if I'm being honest.

Not because I think the world is ending, or because I'm some doomsday pessimist. But because I see what's being normalized. What's being sold to kids as "normal," or "healthy," or "just how things are."

Processed food everywhere. Sedentary lifestyles. Screen addiction. Mental health crises in elementary schools. Kids who can't focus, can't sleep, can't regulate their emotions.

And the systems we're supposed to trust, schools, food companies, even healthcare, they're not designed to make our kids healthy. They're designed to keep them compliant, consuming, and dependent.

That reality doesn't make me hopeless, though. It makes me double down on what I can control.

Because here's the truth: my kids might grow up in a world I can't fix. But I can still make our home a place that builds them up instead of breaking them down.

I can't control what happens out there. But I can absolutely control what happens in here.

And that's where I determine the outcome of the fight.

Feed Their Bodies, Feed Their Future

The easiest and most powerful way to protect your kids' health is to start with their plates.

We live in a time when processed food is cheaper, faster, and more available than organic, chemical-free food. Where a drive-thru meal costs less than a bag of organic vegetables. Where restaurants design kids' menus around what sells, not what nourishes.

And I get it. Life is busy. You're tired. Cooking takes time. It's easier to grab something quickly.

But here's what I've learned raising four kids across different ages: every actual meal you put in front of them is a deposit in their future health account.

All the mangoes from our tree. You can enhance a smoothie with every handful of moringa. Every sweet potato we pull from the ground. Every salad made with greens from the backyard.

Those meals are building their bodies, their brains, their immune systems, their energy levels, their ability to focus, sleep, and regulate their moods.

You're not just feeding them today. You're programming their taste buds, their habits, their relationship with food for the rest of their lives.

Kids don't get to make all their own choices when they're young. But they eat what's put in front of them.

So what are you putting in front of them?

I'm not saying you have to be perfect. We're not perfect. My kids sometimes eat pizza . They have treats. They go to birthday parties and eat cake.

But the foundation, the daily norm, that's actual food. Food we grew or food we know the source of. Food that looks like food, not a science experiment.

And here's the thing: kids adapt faster than you think.

When my oldest was little, we weren't growing food yet. We were buying whatever was convenient. And he grew up thinking chicken nuggets and fries were normal meals.

But when we started the food forest, when fresh fruit and vegetables became the norm, something shifted. His taste buds changed, and so did his energy.

Now he's the one asking for fruit instead of candy. Reaching for water instead of soda.

That didn't happen by accident. It happened because we changed the environment.

And with the younger ones, especially our baby, we have the chance to do it right from the start. To raise a child who never knows processed food as normal. Who grows up eating mangoes off the tree and moringa in smoothies and sweet potatoes fresh from the ground.

That's a gift we can give them that no amount of money can buy.

Make Movement Normal

If kids grow up thinking exercise is punishment, something you do because you're fat or slow or not good enough, they'll avoid it for the rest of their lives.

That's not the relationship I want my kids to have with their bodies.

Around here, movement is just part of life.

We garden together. The older kids helped me move bags of compost and mulch. The younger one's water plants and picks fruit. Everyone works hard.

We ride bikes. We engage in outdoor play. Lifting things is what we do. We run around. We make it fun.

My oldest has trained with me. He's at that age where he wants to get stronger, and instead of just talking about it, we do it together. I showed him how to lift. How to push himself. How to rest and recover.

My middle kids help in the garden and chase each other around the yard until they're exhausted and happy.

And even the baby, barely walking, is outside with us. Crawling through the grass. Touching leaves. Experiencing the world with his whole body, not just his eyes on a screen.

You don't have to force workouts on kids. You don't have to make them run laps or do push-ups as punishment.

You just have to create an environment where their bodies are used to being active. Where movement feels as natural as breathing.

Because when they're older, when you're not there to guide them, that foundation will stay with them.

They won't see exercise as something they "should" do. They'll see it as something they want to do because it feels good, because it's part of who they are.

That's the goal.

Teach them to think for themselves

I want my kids to think for themselves. Not just repeat what they hear on TV, or read online, or learn in school.

I want them to question things. To dig deeper. To ask "why," "how do you know," and "what's the evidence."

That starts young.

When they ask me a question, I don't always give them the answer right away. I asked for their opinions. I teach them how to find the information. I instruct them on evaluating sources, discerning fact from opinion, and critical thinking.

It's not about making them cynical or distrustful. It's about making them sharp.

Because the world is full of people trying to sell them something. Junk food marketed as healthy. Influencers pushing products. News designed to make them scared or angry.

If they can't think for themselves, they'll be easy targets.

But if they can question, research, and think critically, they'll be dangerous. In the best possible way.

Healthy kids aren't just strong in body. They're sharp of mind.

And in a world that profits from keeping people dumb and distracted, raising smart, curious, thoughtful kids is an act of rebellion.

Guard their minds as you guard their health

It's not just junk food that's hurting kids. It's junk information.

Toxic social media. Endless scrolling. Brain-rotting content designed to hook them and keep them coming back for more.

The average kid spends 4-6 hours a day on screens. That's more time than they spend outside, reading, playing, creating, or talking to their family combined.

Think about that.

Their brains are being shaped by algorithms designed to maximize engagement, not growth. By content designed to sell ads, not build character.

And we wonder why anxiety and depression in kids are at all-time highs.

I'm not anti-technology. My kids have access to screens. But it's limited, intentional, and monitored.

Because protecting their mental space is just as important as protecting their physical health.

Our home is a place where conversations matter more than notifications. Where people value books more than trending videos. Where hands-on learning, building things, growing things, and creating things are the norm.

That doesn't happen by accident. It's a choice Toni and I make every day.

And yeah, my kids push back sometimes. They want more screen time. They want to do what their friends are doing.

But I prefer them to feel frustrated now rather than to break later.

Because once social media destroys their attention span, hijacks their dopamine system, and ties their self-worth to likes and followers, it's incredibly hard to undo.

So we set boundaries. We protect their minds. We create space for them to be bored, to imagine, to think, to just be kids.

That's our job as parents. Not to be their friends. Not to give them everything they want. But to protect them from things they're not ready for.

Let the Garden Be Their Classroom

The food forest teaches my kids lessons no textbook can match.

Patience is what they see when a tree takes three years to fruit. They can't rush it. They can't skip the process. It is necessary for them to wait and tend.

They see resilience when a plant gets knocked down by a storm and grows back stronger. They learn setbacks aren't the end of the story.

They see cause and effect when they forget to water something and it dies. Actions have consequences. Neglect has a cost.

They see abundance when one sweet potato slip turns into ten pounds of food. They learn that small, consistent efforts compound into big results.

Every time they plant a seed and watch it grow, they're learning responsibility. Self-reliance. The value of hard work.

And they're learning it not from me lecturing them, but from the plants showing them.

That kind of education sticks. Because they're experiencing it, not just hearing about it.

My older kids now understand that food doesn't come from a store. It comes from soil, sun, water, and time.

They know that if they want fruit; they have to plant a tree and wait.

They know that if they want vegetables; they have to tend the garden.

That knowledge will serve them for the rest of their lives.

And with the baby, I can't wait to see him grow up in a world where this is normal. Where planting food is just what we do. Where dirt under his nails is a sign of a good day.

That's the childhood I want for all of them. Rooted in something real.

Lead by Example (Because Kids Watch Everything)

Here's the hard truth: if I tell my kids to eat healthy, but I'm drinking soda all day, they'll remember what I do, not what I say.

If I tell them to be strong but they never see me train, my words won't mean much.

If I tell them to read but I'm scrolling on my phone all night, they'll follow my actions, not my advice.

Kids watch more than they listen.

They're paying attention to how you live, not just what you preach.

So if you want to raise healthy kids in a sick world, you have to be the healthy adult they can copy.

That's the standard. And it's a high one.

It means I can't just talk about fitness. I have to train. I have to show them what discipline looks like.

It means I can't just talk about eating clean. I have to eat cleanly. I have to model the relationship with food I want them to have.

It means I can't just talk about hard work. I have to work hard in the garden and at the gym. In my business. In my relationship both personal and business.

Because they're watching.

And one day, when I'm not around, when they're making their own choices, they'll fall back on what they saw me do.

That's terrifying and beautiful at the same time.

It makes me want to be better. Not perfect, but better. Consistent. Intentional. Present.

Because I'm not just raising kids. I'm raising future adults. Future parents. Future leaders.

And the example I set now will echo in their lives, and in their kids' lives, long after I'm gone.

That's a legacy. And it's worth fighting for.

The Gift of Hard Things

I'm never going to tell anyone how to raise their kids. Every family is unique. Every situation is unique.

But if there's one piece of advice I'd give, one principle I'd pass on, it's this: don't be afraid to make your kids do hard things.

Hard things build healthy kids.

That might look like helping you move bags of dirt for the garden. Going on a jog together even when they don't feel like it. Waking them up at a set time to do some exercise or chores before the day starts.

It's not punishment. It's training for life.

Because the world is hard. Life is hard. And if your kids never learn how to do hard things when they're young and you're there to support them, life will crush them when they're older and alone.

Doing hard things teaches discipline. Structure. Delayed gratification. Grit. The ability to push through discomfort.

Those are lessons that will carry them further than comfort ever could.

And in a world that makes everything easy, that coddles kids and removes every obstacle, raising children who can handle "hard" is one of the greatest gifts you can give them.

My kids don't always like it at the moment. They complain. Their complaint is noted. They'd rather play video games or watch TV.

But later, when they finish something difficult, when they look back and realize they did it, I see the pride in their eyes.

That's confidence you can't buy. That's strength you can't fake.

And that's what I want for them. Not a simple life. A strong life. Because I know the world will not love my babies as my wife and I do. They will not receive a hug from the world when they make mistakes.

Practical Ways to Start Right Now

If you're reading this and thinking, "Okay, I want this for my kids. Where do I start?" here's what I'd tell you:

1. **Cook with them**

Teach them where food comes from and how to prepare it. Let them crack eggs, stir pots, chop vegetables (age-appropriate, obviously). Make it fun, not a chore.

The kitchen is one of the most important classrooms in your home.

2. **Plant something together**

Even a small pot of herbs can be their responsibility. Allow them to water it. Let them watch it grow. Let them harvest it and use it in a meal.

That simple act teaches so much.

3. Have active family time

Walk together. Ride bikes. Play a sport. Work in the garden. Make movement a thing you do together, not something they do alone or avoid.

The family that moves together stays strung together.

4. Read together

Fill their minds with ideas and stories that inspire them. Not just kids' books (though those are great), but books that challenge them, stretch them, and make them think.

Books build vocabulary, imagination, empathy, and critical thinking. That's a foundation that lasts.

5. Limit the noise

More genuine conversations. Fewer hours of scrolling. More time outside. Less time on screens.

Protect their attention as you protect their health.

6. Let them see you fail and keep going

Don't hide your struggles from them. Let them see you try something, fail, and try again. Let them see you work hard, rest, and come back stronger.

That teaches resilience better than any lecture ever could.

Final Word: Your Home Is a Fortress

The world will not get less complicated. It will not get cleaner, safer, or healthier on its own.

But your home can be a fortress if you build it that way.

A place where actual organic food is normal. This is where movement is an essential part of life. This is a place that protects and nurtures minds. Where people value hard work. Where kids learn to think, grow, create, and thrive.

You can't control the world out there. But you can absolutely control the world in here.

And that makes all the difference.

Feed their bodies real food. Feed their minds with truth and wisdom. Keep their spirits strong by teaching them to do hard things.

Raising healthy kids in a sick world isn't about perfection. It's about consistency.

Every healthy habit you build now is a seed they'll carry into their own future. Every lesson you teach by example is a tool they'll use for the rest of their lives.

You're not just raising children. You're raising the next generation.

And if you do it right, they'll be stronger, smarter, healthier, and more capable than the generation before them.

Pursuing that is our goal. That's the fight. That's the legacy.

So plant the seeds. Do the work. Lead by example.

Your kids are watching. And they're counting on you to show them the way.

Don't let them down.

Chapter 13

PLANTING TREES YOU'LL NEVER CLIMB

Some people think planting a tree is just about fruit.

For me, it's about time. The time I'll never get back and the time I'll never see.

When I put a mango tree in the ground today, I'm not just thinking about the first fruit I'll taste in three years. I'm thinking further. Way further.

I'm thinking about my children. And maybe one day, their kids. Standing under that same tree, picking fruit, completely unaware that their grandfather had planted it decades ago.

I'm thinking about the shade it will give on summer days I'll never experience.

I'm thinking about the fact that my hands started something that will keep giving long after I'm gone.

That's a legacy.

Not a headstone with my name on it. Not money in a bank account. Memories that lose their clarity over time are not even comparable.

But something alive. Something useful. Something that keeps producing, keeps providing, keeps serving people I'll never meet.

That's the legacy I want to leave.

Legacy Is More Than Money

I've seen people leave stacks of money to their family, only for it to be gone in a few years. Spent. Squandered. Fought over. Wasted on things that don't last.

But a food forest? A set of skills? A mindset that knows how to survive and thrive?

People cannot steal, tax, or spend that inheritance.

Money disappears. Habits last. Discipline compounds. A way of life endures through generations.

If my kids grow up knowing how to grow food, care for their bodies, protect their minds, and think for themselves, they'll be rich no matter what's in their bank account.

That's the wealth that matters. The kind that doesn't show up on a balance sheet but shows up in how they live, how they raise their own kids, how they handle hard times.

I can't guarantee they'll have money. The economy could crash. Jobs could disappear. Inflation could destroy savings.

But I can guarantee they'll know how to feed themselves. How to stay strong. Ways to adapt. How to create instead of just consume.

That's the inheritance I'm building. Not for them to spend, but for them to use. To live. To pass on.

What they see is what they learn

Kids rarely remember speeches. But they never forget what they see every day.

If they watch me out in the yard working the land, staying fit, reading, building, they'll remember that as "normal."

They won't think it's special. They'll think it's just what you do. What adults do. What their family does.

And that becomes their baseline. Their standard. Their expectations of themselves.

People don't build legacies with grand gestures. It's built in the quiet hours. Mornings when I'm mulching before sunrise, while most of the neighborhood is still asleep, are quite interesting. The evenings when I'm pruning instead of sitting in front of a screen. The daily choice to do the work even when nobody's clapping for it.

That's what they'll carry with them.

Not the things I said. But the things I did. Over and over. Consistently. Without fanfare.

My oldest has trained with me now. Not because I forced him. But because he's been watching me, do it his whole life. It's normal for him. It's what men in our family do.

My middle children help in the garden without being asked. My babies know how to take care of most things in the garden, which include watering, harvesting, and identifying pests, better than most gardeners.

And our baby boy, barely walking, already reaches for fruit off the trees. Already puts his hands in the soil. Already knows that outside is where life happens.

I didn't sit them down and lecture about any of this. I just lived it. And they absorbed it.

That's how legacy works. It's caught, not taught.

A Food Forest Is a Time Capsule

Every plant in my yard has a story stitched into it.

The pomegranate tree with my wife Toni's placenta buried beneath it. A living marker of new life. A tree that will feed our family for decades, rooted in the literal beginning of our youngest son's life.

The mango tree planted in honor of my father. A reminder of the roots he gave me. Every fruit that tree produces carries its name in my heart.

The moringa I planted after he passed, during those dark months when I didn't know how to move forward. That tree grew while I healed. And now it feeds my family every week.

The lemongrass my wife brought home without knowing I was researching it. God is good!

The elderberry that neighbors have shared for years. Proof that health spreads when you give it away.

Years from now, long after I'm gone, these stories will still be here. Speaking for me when I can't.

My great-grandchildren might not know my voice. They might not remember my face. But they'll stand under these same trees, taste the same fruit, and know somebody cared enough to plant them.

That somebody planted with intention. With love. With hope for a future that they would never see.

That's a message that transcends time.

Legacy Requires Intention

You don't stumble into a legacy. You don't accidentally leave something meaningful behind.

You build it. One intentional choice at a time.

That's why I'm deliberate about what I plant. Not just any tree, but trees that will produce for decades. Trees that are suited to this climate, this soil, this land.

That's why I'm deliberate about what I teach my kids. Not just random information, but skills they can use. Mindsets they can apply. Principles they can build.

That's why I'm deliberate about where I spend my time. Because time is the only resource you can't get back. And how I spend it today determines what I leave behind tomorrow.

Every lesson I give my kids about the garden, every workout they see me finish, every book I put in their hands, every conversation we have around the dinner table, that's a brick in the foundation I'm laying for them.

This isn't about creating a perfect life for them. I can't do that. Life is hard. Challenges will come. Loss will come. Struggle will come.

But I can give them tools. Tools they can use no matter what life throws at them.

The ability to grow food means they'll never go hungry, no matter what the economy does.

The habit of training their body means they'll stay strong as they age.

Reading and thinking critically means my children won't easily let anyone manipulate them. They will question everything.

The foundation of faith means they'll have something to stand on when everything else shakes.

Those tools are my legacy. And I'm placing them in their hands one day at a time.

Planting for People You'll Never Meet

Some trees I plant won't reach their prime until I'm gone.

I'll never taste the fruit. I'll never sit in the full shade. I'll never see them at their peak.

And that's fine.

Actually, it's more than fine. It's the point.

Legacy work isn't about instant payoff. It's not about seeing the results in your lifetime.

It's about faith.

Faith that the work I'm doing today will matter to people I'll never meet.

Faith that a shade tree planted now will give rest to someone else decades from now.

Faith that a piece of land I nurtured will still thrive when my name is just a story passed down.

When I think about my great-grandkids walking these same paths, leaning against these same trees, tasting fruit I never got to try, I realize this isn't just about plants.

This is about people. People I'll love without ever knowing them. People who will benefit from choices I made before they were born.

That's a different reward. Not immediate. Not tangible. But deeply, profoundly meaningful.

I'm planting trees I'll never climb. And I'm okay with that.

Because someone climbed trees, their grandfather planted. And I benefited from work people did before I was born.

That's how it's supposed to work. Each generation plants for the next. Each generation finishes what previous generations left and adds to it.

We're links in a chain. And the strength of that chain depends on whether we do our part.

I'm doing mine.

The Quiet Immortality

We all leave something behind when we're gone.

For some people, it's debt. Bad habits. Broken relationships. Pain that echoes through generations.

For others, it's wisdom. Health. Systems that work. Love that multiplies.

I choose to leave a living inheritance.

When I'm gone, my voice won't echo in their ears anymore. But the systems I've built will still be there.

The garden, producing food year after year.

The gym habits passed down from father to son to grandson.

The love of learning, carried forward in the books they read and the questions they ask.

The faith in God, rooted deeper than any tree.

That's the immortality that matters to me.

Not fame or recognition. Not even being remembered. Although admittedly I want to be remembered as a man who helped people and a man of God. Whoever looks up to me, I want them to see faith, family, fitness, and finance are something I don't take lightly.

But knowing that what I started will continue. That the seeds I planted, literal and metaphorical, will keep growing.

That my great-great-grandkids will eat fruit from trees I planted. Will read the books I collected. Will train their bodies because it's "just what our family does."

They might not know why. They might not know where it started.

But it will still be there. Still working. Still blessing them.

That's a legacy.

This Is Bigger Than Gardening

Let me be clear about something: this book isn't just about gardening.

It's not even just about health, or fitness, or food.

It's about leaving the land better than I found it. Raising my family stronger than I was raised. Making sure that the knowledge, the habits, the hope that kept me going don't die with me.

That's the mission.

Because when I look at the world my kids are growing up in, I see a lot of broken systems. A lot of dependence. Many people are waiting for someone else to save them.

I don't want that for my bloodline.

I want my descendants to be strong. Independent. Capable. Rooted in something real.

I want them to know how to create, not just consume. How to build, not just buy. How to provide, not just hope someone else will.

And that starts now. With the choices I make. The example I set. The systems I build.

The work we do in our gardens, in our gyms, in our homes, in our libraries, it's not just for now.

It's for every generation that comes after us.

Every tree planted is a gift to the future.

Every workout completed is a deposit in the health of your lineage.

By reading every book, one gains wisdom to pass down.

Every meal grown and shared is a lesson in self-reliance.

This is legacy work. And it's the most important work you'll ever do.

What will you leave behind?

Here's the question I want you to sit with: What are you leaving behind?

If you died tomorrow, what would your kids inherit from you?

Not your stuff. Anyone can leave stuff.

But what skills would they have because you taught them? What habits would they carry because they watched you live them? What systems would still produce because you built them?

What trees would still grow?

That's the standard. That's the bar.

And I know it's high. I know it's hard.

But it's worth it.

Because the alternative is leaving nothing. Or worse, leaving debt, dysfunction, and dependence.

I refuse to do that to my family.

So I plant. I build. I teach. I train. I lead.

Not perfectly. Not always successfully. But consistently. Intentionally.

My eyes are on a future I'll never see, but my hands are working to create it, anyway.

That's a legacy.

And it starts today. With one seed. A single workout. One lesson. One choice.

What will you plant today that will still grow when you're gone?

That's the question. And the answer is up to you.

But I'll tell you this: the best time to plant a tree was twenty years ago.

The second-best time is right now.

So get to work.

Plant something that outlives you.

Build something that serves people you'll never meet.

Leave the land, the family, the world, better than you found it.

That's the calling.

That's the legacy.
Now go live it.

Chapter 14

THE FLORIDA SURVIVOR FIFTEEN

Florida isn't a state that forgives mistakes.

Plant tomatoes in July and watch them wilt. Put a mango in a low spot and it'll drown in the wet season. Forget to mulch, and your plants will bake in the sun.

This state will humble you fast if you don't know what you're doing.

But here's the flip side: the right plant in the right place, planted at the right time, will not only survive, it will thrive.

These fifteen plants are my proven staples. I've planted them. Grown them. Eaten them. Relied on them when money was tight and food prices went wild.

This isn't theory. This works in Zones 9-11, tested in West Central Florida heat, sandy soil, afternoon thunderstorms, and the occasional hurricane.

Below, I'll show you exactly where to put them, when to plant them, what they taste like, how to use them in your kitchen, and how to keep them alive through everything Florida throws at you.

No fluff. Just what works.

This updated edition will include notation of plants that survived the cold in Central Florida, as well as those that proved difficult for most backyard growers below 32 degrees for 3-4 consecutive nights.

Let's get into it.

Moringa (Moringa oleifera)

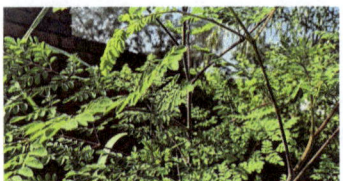
Moringa

The Multivitamin Tree

Zones: 9-11 (dies back in freezes but regrows from roots in zone 9) **Cold sensitive. Needs frost protection or to be brought indoors when temperatures drop to 32 degrees or below.**

When to Plant: Spring through summer, once nighttime temperatures stay consistently above 60°F. In South Florida, you can plant year-round.

Soil Requirements: Sandy or loamy soil that drains fast. Moringa hates to sit in water. If you've got a low spot that floods, plant on a mound or don't plant it there at all.

What It Tastes Like: Fresh young leaves taste like a spicy cross between spinach and horseradish, with a mustard-green kick. Cooked, they mellow out to a rich, earthy green that works in soups and stir-fries. The pods (drumsticks) taste like green beans with a nutty twist.

How to Grow It:

Full sun is non-negotiable. Moringa in the shade is a waste of space.

Plant trees 6 to 10 feet apart. If you're planting multiple, give them room.

Here's the key: prune hard and prune often. I'm talking aggressively. Cut it back to 3-4 feet every 2-3 months. If you don't, it'll grow into a tall, skinny telephone pole with all the leaves out of reach.

Every time you prune, it bushes out and produces more tender growth at picking height. That's what you want.

Water young trees 2-3 times per week until established. Once they're 6-8 months old, they're drought tolerant and thrive on neglect.

Pests/Problems: pest-free. Occasionally aphids or caterpillars, but nothing serious.

How to Use It:

- Add fresh young leaves to salads (use sparingly, they're strong)
- Cook leaves like spinach in soups, stews, or stir-fries
- Dry and grind leaves into powder for smoothies, teas, or sprinkling over rice
- Flowers make a light, fragrant tea
- Steam young pods like green beans for curries and soups

Why It's a Survivor: Fast-growing, nutrient-dense, produces year-round in South Florida, handles poor soil, drought-tolerant once established, and is nearly impossible to kill.

Sweet Potato (Ipomoea batatas)

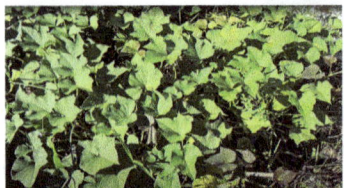

Sweet Potato

The Underground Workhorse

Zones: 8-11. **Cold sensitive. Needs frost protection or to be brought indoors when temperatures drop to 32 degrees or below**.

When to Plant: March through June for a summer/fall harvest. You can plant again in August for a late fall crop if you're in South Florida.

Soil Requirements: Loose, sandy soil is perfect. Sweet potatoes love Florida's sand if you amend it with compost. Raised beds or mounds work best because they need good drainage.

What it tastes like: The roots are sweet, earthy, and creamy when roasted. Young leaves (the greens) taste like spinach with a nutty undertone and are completely edible.

How to Grow It:

Start with slips (rooted cuttings from a sweet potato). You can buy them or make your own by suspending a sweet potato in water until it sprouts.

Plant slips on 12-inch-high mounds, spaced 12-18 inches apart. The mounds improve drainage and make harvesting easier.

Water regularly for the first month until vines run. Once established, sweet potatoes are incredibly drought-tolerant.

The vines will sprawl and smother weeds. Let them.

Harvest 90-120 days after planting, when the leaves yellow. Don't wait too long, or critters will find them first.

Pests/Problems: Occasional deer or armadillo damage. Wireworms if the soil is too wet.

How to Use It:

- Roast whole or cubed with olive oil and herbs
- Mash for pies, casseroles, or as a side dish
- Stir-fry the young leaves (called sweet potato greens) with garlic
- Slice thin and bake as chips
- Add to soups and stews

Why It's a Survivor: One slip produces 5-10 pounds of food. Handles poor soil. Thrives in heat. Stores for months. Provides both roots and greens. This is a high-calorie, high-return crop.

Katuk (Sauropus androgynus)

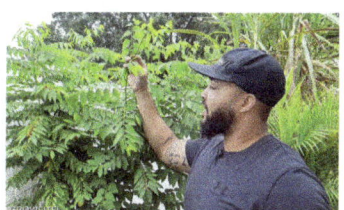

Katuk

The Shade-Loving Green Machine

Zones: 9-11. **Cold-sensitive. Needs frost protection or to be brought indoors when temperatures drop to 32 degrees or below.**

When to Plant: Spring through summer, once the soil warms up.

Soil Requirements: Rich, moist soil with good drainage. Add compost before planting.

What it tastes like? : Fresh leaves are crunchy with a flavor like green peas mixed with peanuts. Unique and addictive.

How to Grow It:

This is one of the few productive greens that actually prefers partial shade. Plant it under the canopy of fruit trees, along fences, or on the north side of structures.

Space plants 3 feet apart if you're creating a hedge.

Pinch the growing tips often to keep plants short, bushy, and productive. If you let it grow tall without pruning, it'll get leggy.

Keep it watered during dry spells and heat waves. Mulch heavily.

Pests/Problems: Mostly pest-free. Occasionally aphids.

How to Use It:

- Eat raw leaves as a snack straight off the bush
- Toss into salads for a nutty crunch
- Blanch lightly and serve with rice
- Add to soups at the end of cooking
- Brew dried leaves for a mild tea

Why It's a Survivor: Grows in shade where most productive plants won't. Produces year-round. Low maintenance. High in protein for a leafy green. Kids actually like eating it because it tastes good raw.

Pigeon pea (Cajanus cajan)

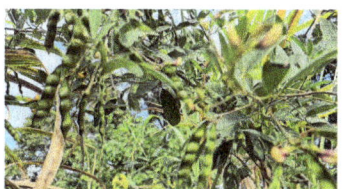
Pigeon Pea Plant

The nitrogen-fixing permaculture staple

Zones: 9-11. **Cold sensitive. Needs frost protection or to be brought indoors when temperatures drop to 32 degrees or below.**

When to Plant: Spring through early summer.

Soil Requirements: Tolerates sandy, rocky, and poor soils better than almost anything else. Doesn't need amendments.

What It Tastes Like: Fresh beans taste like a cross between lentils and peas with a nutty, earthy flavor. Dried beans are heartier and meatier.

How to Grow It:

Directly sow seeds 1 inch deep, 4-6 feet apart. They'll grow into 6-10 foot shrubs in a matter of months.

Pigeon peas fix nitrogen in the soil, so they actually improve fertility while producing food. That's why they're a permaculture favorite.

They also work as windbreaks, nurse plants for young fruit trees, and chop-and-drop mulch sources.

Water until established. After that, they thrive on neglect.

Pests/Problems: Mostly pest-free. Occasionally pod borers.

How to Use It:

- Boil fresh green peas and season them like any bean
- Dry mature beans for long-term storage
- Cook dried beans into hearty soups, stews, or rice and peas

- Use leaves as mulch or compost material
- Brew leaves as a medicinal tea (traditionally used for respiratory issues)

Why It's a Survivor: Fixes nitrogen. Tolerates poor soil. Drought-tolerant. Produces protein-rich food. Reseeds itself. Serves multiple functions in a food forest system.

Everglades Tomato (Solanum pimpinellifolium)

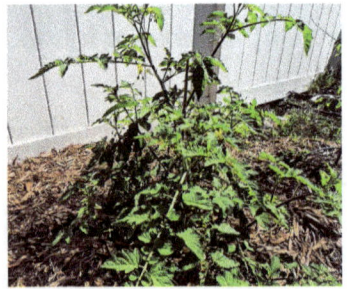

Everglades Tomato Plant

The Florida Heat Champion

Zones: 9-11. **Cold-tolerant. Can handle temperatures at or below 32 degrees for short periods without protection.**

When to Plant: Spring and summer, especially when traditional tomatoes are dying in the heat.

Soil Requirements: Thrives in sandy, poor soil. Doesn't need heavy amendments.

What It Tastes Like: Marble-sized cherry tomatoes that are intensely sweet-tart and burst with flavor. Way more flavor than grocery store tomatoes.

How to Grow It:

Scatter seeds in prepared beds or let them self-sow. Water lightly until sprouts appear.

Let the vines sprawl on the ground or climb fences. They're semi-wild and don't need staking like traditional tomatoes.

This variety handles Florida's heat and humidity without getting the diseases that kill regular tomatoes in summer.

It reseeds prolifically. Once you plant it, you'll have volunteers every year.

Pests/Problems: Hornworms occasionally. More resistant to pests and diseases than regular tomatoes.

How to Use It:

- Eat fresh, right off the vine
- Toss into salads for bursts of flavor
- Roast and blend into sauces
- Halve and dry for sun-dried tomatoes
- Ferment for hot sauce

Why It's a Survivor: Handles heat that kills other tomatoes. Disease-resistant. Reseeds itself. Produces when nothing else will. This is the tomato that actually works in Florida summers.

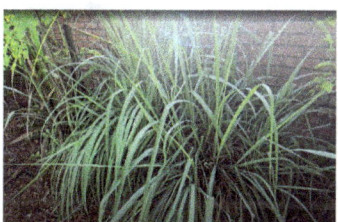

Lemongrass

Lemongrass (Cymbopogon citratus)

The Kitchen and Medicine Cabinet Staple

Zones: 9-11. **Cold-tolerant. Can handle temperatures at or below 32 degrees for short periods without protection.**

When to Plant: Spring through summer.

Soil Requirements: Thrives in sandy, well-drained soil. Tolerates poor soil if mulched.

What it tastes like: Fresh citrus flavor with lemon and mint notes. Aromatic and refreshing.

How to Grow It:

Plant clumps (divisions from an existing plant) 2-3 feet apart in full sun.

Water regularly to establish. Once established, it's fairly drought-tolerant but appreciates consistent moisture.

Divide clumps every year or two. One plant becomes 5-10 plants quickly.

Pests/Problems: Virtually pest-free.

How to Use It:

- Chop white inner stalks for stir-fries, curries, and marinades (Southeast Asian cuisine staple)

- Brew leaves and stalks into tea for digestion, relaxation, and immune support

- Use whole stalks to flavor soups and broths (remove before serving)

- Dry and grind for spice blends

Why It's a Survivor: Low-maintenance. Pest-free. Multiplies freely. Dual-purpose (culinary and medicinal). Produces year-round. This is a plant every Florida garden needs.

Banana (Musa spp.)

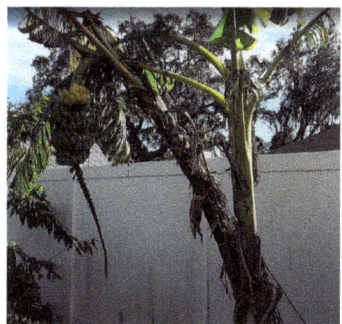
Banana Plant

The Fast-Producing Tropical Staple

Zones: 9-11 (some cold-hardy varieties tolerate zone 8 with protection)

Cold sensitive. Needs frost protection or to be brought indoors when temperatures drop to 32 degrees or below.

When to plant: Anytime the soil is warm, ideally in spring.

Soil Requirements: Loves rich, moist soil with lots of organic matter. Heavy feeder.

What it tastes like: Varies by variety. 'Apple Banana' has a tangy, apple-like flavor. 'Ice Cream' (Blue Java) tastes like vanilla ice cream. 'Cavendish' is the standard grocery store flavor.

How to Grow It:

Dig a banana circle: a 6-8 foot wide depression filled with organic waste (kitchen scraps, yard waste, coffee grounds). Plant pups around the rim.

Bananas are heavy feeders and water lovers. Keep them well-watered and fed with compost.

Manage each mat to have one mother (producing), one child (next to produce), and one grandchild (coming up). Remove extra pups and plant elsewhere or give them away.

After a plant fruits, it dies. Cut it down and let the next generation take over.

Pests/Problems: Nematodes in some areas. Panama disease (Fusarium wilt) is a concern for certain varieties. Choose resistant varieties if available.

How to Use It:
- Eat ripe fruit raw or in smoothies
- Fry green bananas for tostones or chips
- Bake or boil green bananas as a starchy side
- Wrap fish, meat, or tamales in banana leaves for steaming
- Use leaves as biodegradable plates

Why It's a Survivor: Produces fruit in 9-18 months. Constant production with proper mat management. Handles Florida's wet season. Multiple uses (fruit, leaves, fiber). High-calorie food sources.

Mulberry (Morus spp.)

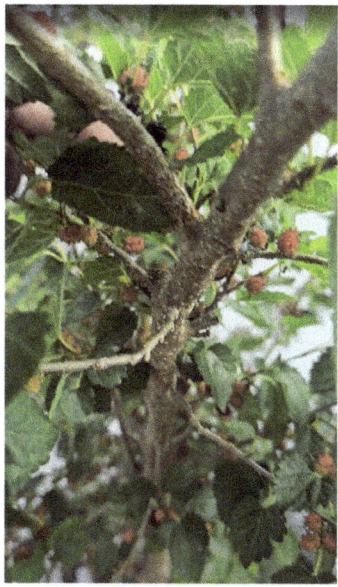
Everbearing Mulberry Tree

The Easy, Abundant Fruit Tree

Zones: 8-11. **Cold tolerant. Can handle temperatures at or below 32 degrees for short periods without protection**.

When to Plant: Early spring or fall for best establishment.

Soil Requirements: Adaptable to most soils. Prefers rich, loamy soil but tolerates sand and clay.

What it tastes like: Sweet, juicy berries with a blackberry-like flavor. Some varieties are sweeter than others.

How to Grow It:

Plant in full sun, 15-20 feet apart. These trees grow big.

Prune after fruiting to keep the tree low and manageable. If you let it grow tall, you'll be feeding birds instead of yourself.

Mulberries are incredibly low-maintenance. Water young trees until established; then they handle drought well.

Pests/Problems: Birds love them. Net the tree or plant enough to share. Fruit stains everything, so don't plant over driveways or patios.

How to Use It:

- Eat fresh by the handful (kids love them)
- Blend into smoothies, jams, or syrups
- Bake into pies, muffins, and cobblers
- Dry for long-term storage
- Ferment into wine

Why It's a Survivor: Produces heavily with zero care. Tolerates neglect. No major pest or disease issues in Florida. Fruit ripens over several weeks, giving you a long harvest window.

Barbados Cherry (Malpighia emarginata)

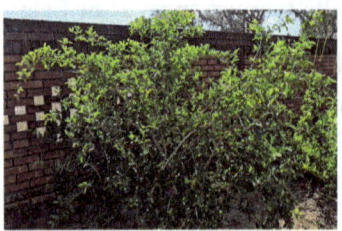

Barbados Cherry Tree

The Vitamin C Powerhouse

Zones: 9-11. **Cold sensitive. Needs frost protection or to be brought indoors when temperatures drop to 32 degrees or below.**

When to plant: Spring or summer.

Soil Requirements: Well-drained sandy soil enriched with compost. Does not tolerate wet feet.

What it tastes like: Tart-sweet cherries with an intense, tangy flavor. One of the highest natural sources of vitamin C on the planet.

How to Grow It:

Plant in full sun for maximum production. Space 8 to 10 feet apart.

Mulch heavily and water deeply during dry periods. Once established, it's fairly drought-tolerant but produces better with consistent moisture.

Light pruning after harvest encourages bushier growth and more fruiting.

Pests/Problems: Relatively pest-free. Fruit flies occasionally appear in the wet season.

How to Use It:

- Juice fresh for vitamin-packed drinks (extremely high in vitamin C)
- Blend into smoothies
- Eat fresh (very tart, not everyone's preference raw)
- Make into jelly, syrup, or preserves
- Freeze for long-term storage

Why It's a Survivor: Produces multiple flushes of fruit per year. Extremely high nutritional value. Handles Florida heat. Low maintenance once established.

Guava (Psidium guajava)

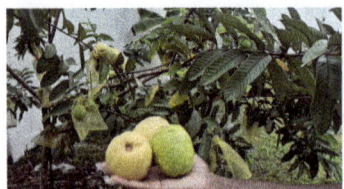

Guava Tree - Ruby Supreme

The Tropical Flavor Bomb

Zones: 9-11. **Cold sensitive. Needs frost protection or to be brought indoors when temperatures drop to 32 degrees or below.**

When to Plant: Spring or early summer.

Soil Requirements: Sandy, well-drained soil. Tolerates poor soil but produces better with compost.

What it tastes like: Sweet, tropical, floral fruit with a custard-like texture. The seeds are edible. Flavor varies by variety from strawberry-like to musky.

How to Grow It:

Plant on a mound in full sun. Space 12 to 15 feet apart.

Bagging fruit (putting paper or fabric bags over developing fruit) protects from fruit flies. This is worth the effort.

Prune to keep the tree at a manageable height. Guavas fruit on recent growth, so annual pruning actually increases production.

Pests/Problems: Fruit flies are the main issue. Caribbean fruit flies will ruin your harvest if you don't bag or time your harvest right.

How to Use It:

- Eat fresh with a sprinkle of salt (classic)

- Blend into juice, smoothies, or agua fresca

- Make guava paste (dulce de guayaba)

- Use in pastries, empanadas, or BBQ sauces

- Dehydrate slices for fruit leather

Why It's a Survivor: Highly productive. Handles poor soil. Drought-tolerant once established. Multiple uses. High vitamin C content. Fruits twice a year in Florida.

Passion Fruit(Passiflora edulis)

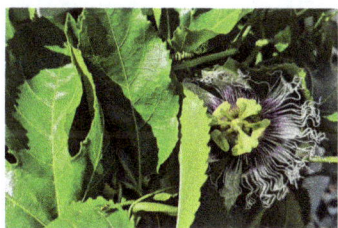

Passion Fruit

The Aromatic Vine Crop

Zones: 9-11. **Cold sensitive. Needs frost protection or to be brought indoors when temperatures drop to 32 degrees or below**.

When to Plant: Spring or early summer.

Soil Requirements: Fertile, well-drained soil. Benefits from compost and mulch.

What it tastes like: Intensely aromatic, sweet-tart pulp with edible seeds. Tropical and exotic flavors.

How to Grow It:

Train vines on trellises, fences, or arbors. They're vigorous climbers and need support.

Water consistently, especially during flowering and fruiting.

Vines are short-lived in Florida (2-4 years). Plan to replace them when production drops.

Pests/Problems: Fungal issues in the wet season. Caterpillars occasionally. Root rot if drainage is poor.

How to Use It:

- Scoop pulp and eat fresh (seeds included)
- Mix into juice, lemonade, or cocktails
- Blend into desserts, ice cream, or yogurt
- Use in sauces, glazes, or salad dressings
- Strain the pulp for smooth juice or syrup.

Why It's a Survivor: High-value crop (expensive to buy). Produces heavily in a small space. Vertical growing saves ground space. Incredibly flavorful.

Sugarcane (Saccharum officinarum)

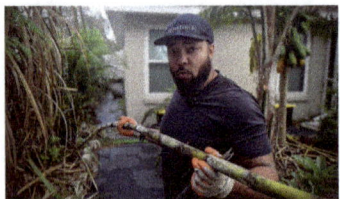

Sugarcane

The Natural Sweetener

Zones: 9-11. **Cold tolerant. Can handle temperatures at or below 32 degrees for short periods without protection.**

When to plant: Early spring or fall.

Soil Requirements: Moist, heavy soil. Great for low spots that stay wet. Tolerates poor drainage better than most crops.

What it tastes like: Sweet, grassy juice with a clean sugarcane flavor. Fresh-pressed juice is incomparable to processed sugar.

How to Grow It:

Lay cuttings (with nodes) in shallow trenches, nodes facing up. Cover with 2 to 3 inches of soil.

Space rows 3 feet apart. Canes grow 8 to 12 feet tall.

Water consistently. Sugarcane loves water and heat.

Harvest after 12-18 months when stalks are thick and mature.

Pests/Problems: Rats and raccoons love sugarcane. Protect harvest.

How to Use It:

- Chew raw stalks for juice (peel the outer layer first)
- Press into fresh cane juice (requires a press or heavy mallet)
- Boil juice down to make syrup or raw sugar
- Use as a natural sweetener in recipes

Why It's a Survivor: Handles wet soil. High-calorie crops. Natural sweetener you control. Handles Florida heat perfectly.

Seminole Pumpkin (Cucurbita moschata)

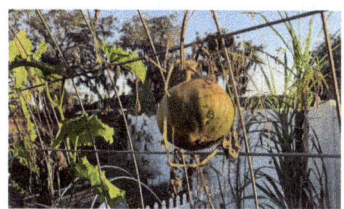

Seminole Pumpkin

The Native Florida Squash

Zones: 8-11. **Cold tolerant. Can handle temperatures at or below 32 degrees for short periods without protection.**

When to plant: Spring or late summer. Avoid planting in peak heat.

Soil Requirements: Sandy, fertile soil amended with compost. Loves mounds.

What it tastes like: Sweet, nutty flesh similar to butternut squash. Dense and flavorful.

How to Grow It:

Plant on compost-enriched mounds. Give vines room to sprawl (15-20 feet).

Hand-pollinate if bees are scarce. Use a paintbrush to transfer pollen from male flowers to female flowers (the ones with small fruit at the base).

Vines are incredibly vigorous. They'll climb trees and fences if you let them.

Pests/Problems: Squash vine borers. Plant early or late to avoid peak borer season. Powdery mildew in humid conditions.

How to Use It:

- Roast flesh like butternut squash
- Blend into soups, stews, or curries
- Bake into pies or bread
- Roast seeds as snacks
- Store whole for months in a cool, dry place

Why It's a Survivor: Native to Florida, adapted to our climate. Handles heat, humidity, and poor soil. Stores for 6+ months. High-calorie food. This is the squash for Florida.

Peanut (Arachis hypogaea)

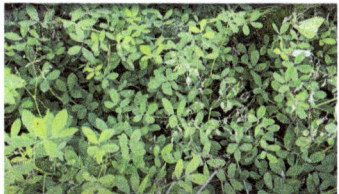

Peanut plant

The Underground Protein Source

Zones: 8-11. **Cold tolerant. Can handle temperatures at or below 32 degrees for short periods without protection**.

When to plant: Late spring to early summer, once the soil is warm.

Soil Requirements: Loose, sandy soil is ideal. Peanuts need loose soil to form pods underground.

What it tastes like: earthy, nutty, rich when roasted. Fresh-dug peanuts are sweeter and more flavorful than store-bought ones .

How to Grow It:

Plant raw, shelled peanuts 1-2 inches deep, 6 inches apart.

Keep soil loose. Don't compact it.

Water consistently, but don't over-water. Peanuts don't like wet feet.

Harvest 120-150 days after planting, when leaves yellow. Dig up the whole plant and shake off the soil. Peanuts will cling to the roots.

Pests/Problems: Nematodes. Rotate crops. Don't plant peanuts in the same spot year after year.

How to Use It:

- Roast for snacks (dry in the sun for a week first, then roast)

- Grind into peanut butter
- Boil fresh peanuts (Southern classic)
- Add to stews, rice dishes, or stir-fries

Why It's a Survivor: High protein. High calories. Fixes nitrogen in the soil. Stores well. Cheap to start (just buy raw peanuts from the store).

Aloe Vera (Aloe barbadensis miller)

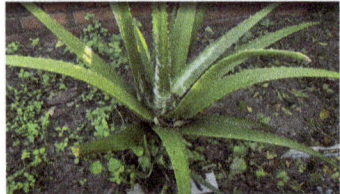

Aloe Vera

The Living First Aid Kit

Zones: 9-11. **Cold tolerant. Can handle temperatures at or below 32 degrees for short periods without protection.**

When to plant: Spring or summer.

Soil Requirements: Sandy, dry, well-drained soil. Hates wet conditions. Perfect for containers.

What it tastes like: The gel is cooling, mildly bitter, and slightly slimy. Mostly used medicinally, not culinarily.

How to Grow It:

Perfect for pots or sandy areas. Needs excellent drainage.

Water deeply, then let the soil dry out completely before watering again. Over-watering kills more aloe than anything else.

Full sun to partial shade. More sun = thicker leaves.

Produces "pups" (baby plants) around the base. Divide and replant.

Pests/Problems: Root rot from over-watering. Scale insects occasionally.

How to Use It:

- Slice leaves and apply gel directly to burns, cuts, or skin irritations
- Blend small amounts of inner gel (not the latex) into smoothies for digestive support (use caution and start small)
- Use in homemade skin and hair care products

Why It's a Survivor: Drought-tolerant. Low maintenance. First aid is always available. Multiplies easily. Thrives in conditions that kill other plants.

Final Thoughts: Build Your System

These fifteen plants form the foundation of a resilient Florida food forest.

They're not the only plants you can grow. But they're the ones I'd bet on if I had to start over from scratch.

Handling Florida's challenges is what they do. They are reliable producers. They serve multiple functions. And they don't require perfection.

Start with three to five from this list. Get them established. Learn their rhythms. Then add more.

Build your system one plant at a time. And in a few years, you'll have a yard that feeds you year-round, no matter what's happening at the grocery store.

That's the goal. This is what freedom is. That's what works in Florida.

Now go plant something.

Chapter 15

EVERYDAY WARRIOR

Not everybody wants to be a bodybuilder.

Not everybody's training for a marathon or trying to set a personal record in the gym.

But everybody needs strength, endurance, and mobility to handle real life.

I call it being an everyday warrior.

You might not be on a battlefield, but life will throw you challenges that demand a powerful body.

Hauling sandbags during hurricane prep. Moving bags of mulch in 95-degree heat. Carrying your kids when they're tired and don't want to walk anymore. Lifting a couch when you're helping a friend move. Cleaning up fallen branches after a storm. Getting down on the floor to play with your grandkids and actually being able to get back up.

If your body's not ready, those moments turn into struggles. Or worse, injuries.

But if you've been training, if you've built real-world strength, those challenges become just another day. No drama. No hesitation. Just handle it and move on.

That's what everyday warrior training is about.

It's not looking great for the beach, which is a nice benefit. I'm not impressing anyone at the gym. I'm not pursuing some idealized aesthetic.

It's about being ready for whatever life throws at you. Today. Tomorrow. Twenty years from now.

It's about building a body that works when you need it to.

Why Everyday Strength Matters?

Your body is the first tool you ever owned, and it's the one you'll use every day until your last breath.

In the garden, in the house, at work, everything's easier when you're stronger. Everything's harder when you're not.

You don't have to deadlift 500 pounds. You don't need to bench press your body weight or run a sub-6-minute mile.

But you should be able to:

- Carry your groceries in one trip without your arms shaking
- Move a wheelbarrow full of soil without blowing out your back
- Pick up a 50-pound bag of compost and load it into your truck
- Get down on the ground and back up without using your hands
- Climb a ladder without your legs trembling
- Work in the yard for a few hours without being wrecked for the next two days

These aren't gym goals. These are life goals.

And the gap between where most people are and where they need to be is bigger than they think.

I see it all the time. People in their 40s and 50s who can't bend over to tie their shoes without their back hurting. Who can't carry a case of water from the car to the house without getting winded. Who avoid physical work because they know their body can't handle it.

That's not aging. That's neglect.

Because I've also seen people in their 60s and 70s who are strong, mobile, and capable. Who can outwork people half their age. Who aren't afraid of physical challenges because they've been training their whole lives.

The difference isn't genetics. It's habits.

You build strength by lifting things.

You maintain mobility by moving through full ranges of motion.

You develop endurance by challenging your cardiovascular system.

Do those things consistently, and your body stays capable. Skip them, and your body breaks down.

It's that simple.

Functional Training, Florida Style

I do not separate my training from my life. It's integrated into it.

The gym keeps me strong. The garden keeps me moving in real-world ways.

And the combination of both creates functional fitness that actually translates to the things I do every day.

Here's how gym movements connect to real life in Florida:

Farmer's Carries (walking while holding heavy weights) → Carrying compost buckets from the pile to the garden. Hauling water jugs during a power outage. Moving sandbags when a hurricane's coming.

Squats and Lunges → Planting. Weeding. Harvesting low-growing crops. Bending down hundreds of times a day in the garden without your knees or back giving out.

Overhead Presses → Pruning fruit trees. Lifting branches. Hanging things. Reaching overhead without shoulder pain.

Deadlifts and Hinges → Picking up bags of soil. Lifting heavy pots. Proper lifting mechanics that protect your back.

Core Work (planks, carries, anti-rotation exercises) → Stability while digging, raking, pushing a wheelbarrow, or carrying uneven loads. A strong core protects your spine during every physical task.

Pull-Ups and Rows → Pulling weeds. Hauling rope. Climbing. Carrying heavy loads in front of your body.

If your workouts don't translate into real-life strength, you're missing the point.

The goal isn't to look like you can work. It's actually to be able to do the work.

Train for consistency, not perfection

Everyday warriors don't train for one big event. They don't peak for a competition or a race.

They train so they're ready every single day. No matter what comes up.

That means no "all or nothing" approach. No waiting for the perfect workout plan or the perfect time to start.

You don't need two hours a day. You need 15-30 minutes consistently.

Some days, I focus on a gym session. An hour of hard work in the yard is what some days entail. Some days it's both.

The key is not letting days pile up without movement.

Because here's what happens when you skip: your body adapts to inactivity. You get weaker. You get stiffer. And when you finally do need your body to perform, it's not ready.

Consistency beats intensity. Every time.

I'd rather see you do 20 minutes of solid work every day than crush yourself for two hours once a week and then do nothing for the next six days.

Build the habit. Show up. Move your body. The strength will come.

Sample Everyday Warrior Routine (20-30 minutes)

This is a simple, effective routine you can do at home with minimal equipment. A pair of dumbbells, a pull-up bar, and your body weight are all you need.

Do this 3-4 times per week. On the other days, work in your garden, go for a walk, or do active recovery.

Warm-up (3-5 minutes)

Get your body ready to move. Don't skip this.

- Jump rope or brisk walk (1-2 minutes)

- Arm circles forward and backward (10 each direction)

- Hip rotations and leg swings (10 each leg)

- Bodyweight squats (10 reps, slow and controlled)

Strength Circuit (Repeat 3 Rounds)

Move through these exercises with minimal rest. Rest 60-90 seconds between rounds.

1. Farmer's Carries - 40-60 feet (grab heavy dumbbells, kettlebells, or even buckets filled with sand/water and walk)

2. Goblet Squats - 15 reps (hold a dumbbell or kettlebell at chest height, squat deep, stand up)

3. Overhead Press - 10 reps each arm (press a dumbbell overhead, control the descent)

4. Plank Hold - 30-60 seconds (keep your body straight, don't let your hips sag)

5. Reverse Lunges- 10 reps each leg (step back, lower your back knee toward the ground, push back up)

Finisher (2-3 minutes)

Push hard for a few minutes to build work capacity and mental toughness.

Pick one:

- Sled pushes (if you have access to a sled)
- Battle ropes (if you have them)
- Wheelbarrow sprints (load it with weight and push it fast)
- Burpees (20-30 reps as fast as you can with excellent form)
- Hill sprints or stair runs

Cool Down (3-5 minutes)

Don't skip this either. Your body needs to recover.

- Walk slowly to bring your heart rate down
- Stretch major muscle groups (hamstrings, quads, chest, shoulders)
- Deep breathing (5-10 deep breaths, in through the nose, out through the mouth)

Notes on the routine:

This simplicity is intentional. That's intentional. You don't need fancy exercises or complex programming.

You need to get stronger at fundamental human movements. Squatting. Hinging. Pushing. Pulling. Carrying. Walking.

Do those things consistently, progressively adding weight or reps over time, and you'll build real-world strength that translates to everything you do.

Scaling the Workout

If you're a beginner:

- Cut the rounds down to 2 instead of 3
- Use lighter weights or bodyweight only
- Take longer rest periods (90-120 seconds between rounds)
- Skip the finisher until you build up work capacity

If you're more advanced:

- Add a fourth round
- Use heavier weights
- Shorten rest periods (30-45 seconds between rounds)
- Add a weighted vest for carries and bodyweight movements
- Make the finisher longer or more intense

The goal is to challenge yourself without breaking yourself. You should finish the workout feeling worked but not destroyed.

Progressive Overload: The Key to Getting Stronger

Here's the secret to building strength over time: progressive overload.

That means you gradually increase the demands on your body. A greater amount of weight. More reps. More rounds. Shorter rest. Whatever variable you choose, you make it slightly harder.

Your body adapts to stress. If you do the same workout with the same weight for months, you'll maintain, but you won't improve.

But if you add 5 pounds to your farmer's carry every few weeks, if you add one more rep to your squats, if you hold your plank 10 seconds longer, your body has to adapt. It gets stronger.

Track your workouts. Write what you did. Next time, try to do a little more.

That's how you build real, lasting strength.

Mindset: The Warrior's Edge

The everyday warrior isn't the strongest person in the room. They're not the fastest or the most athletic.

They're the ones who show up no matter what.

That's the mindset I bring from my garden into my workouts and from my workouts into my life.

Storm hits? I'm ready to clear debris. Not just physically, but mentally. I don't panic. I don't wait for anyone else. I handle it.

Kids need lifting? No problem. My back's strong. My grip's solid. I can carry them as long as they need me to .

Mulch delivery in the heat? Let's go. I've trained in worse. I know my body can handle it.

When you train for life, life doesn't scare you.

You don't avoid physical challenges because you're worried your body will break. You don't hesitate when something heavy needs moving or when work needs doing.

You just do it. Because you know you can.

That confidence, that capability, that's what training gives you.

Not just a powerful body. A powerful mind. A belief that you can handle what comes.

And that's the warrior's edge.

Why I Included Two Training Plans in This Book

And yes, I know I slipped in not one but two training plans in this book.

That's because I love to train. It has shaped my life in ways I can't fully put into words. And I know, deeply, how much it matters.

Some of you might close this book and decide a whole food forest is too much for right now. Maybe you'll start with just a few medicinal herbs on the windowsill, and that's perfectly fine. That's where you should start if that's what you can handle.

But since you're not out there carrying soil bags, digging holes, or planting rows of trees, these workouts will give you a way to move your body and start building actual strength.

Because whether you're gardening, you still need to be strong.

You still need to train your body.

You still need to move.

You still need to prepare for the physical demands life will throw at you.

So even if the garden isn't your thing yet, make the gym (or your garage, or your backyard) your thing.

Start there. Develop strength. Build confidence. Build the body you need to live the life you want.

And maybe, once you feel what it's like to be strong, once you experience the clarity and energy that comes from moving your body consistently, you'll be ready to take on the garden too.

That's the hope, anyway.

A Word of Caution (and Common Sense)

Before you dive into any training program, take care of yourself wisely.

Get a checkup. Talk to your doctor. Make sure you're cleared for exercise, especially if you're over 40, have any chronic health conditions, or haven't been active in a while.

I am not a medical professional. I'm not a certified trainer. I'm just a guy who's been training for years and knows what works for me.

But your body is different. Your history is unique. Your current fitness level is different.

So be smart. Start where you are, not where you think you should be. Listen to your body. If something hurts (not "this is hard" discomfort, but actual pain), stop and figure out what's wrong.

Ego lifting, pushing through injuries, and ignoring warning signs is how people get hurt.

And getting hurt sets you back further than taking it slow ever would.

Be smart about your training. Train consistently. Train for the long haul.

Because this isn't about one workout. It's about building a body that serves you for decades.

Final Word: GrowFit means both

GrowFitFL isn't just about growing food. It's about growing you.

Your strength.

Your health.

Your capability.

Your confidence.

The garden grows your food and your patience. The gym grows your body and your discipline.

Together, they create a complete system. A way of living that makes you resilient, capable, and free.

The everyday warrior builds a body that can work, protect, provide, and play without hesitation.

A body that doesn't quit when things get hard. A body that's ready for whatever comes.

Train as if your future depends on it.

Because it does.

Now let's train.

Chapter 16

SIDE HUSTLE ROOTS

Growing food is powerful.

But growing income from what you love? That takes it to another level.

When you can put food on your table and money in your pocket from the same skills, the same land, the same work you're already doing, you're no longer just gardening.

You're building freedom.

Real freedom. The kind that doesn't depend on a job you hate or a paycheck that barely covers the bills.

I'm not talking about some "get rich quick" nonsense. I will not sell you a dream about quitting your job in 90 days or making six figures from your backyard.

I'm talking about real, steady side income that fits your lifestyle and builds.

Earnings derived from abilities you possess or can gain. Income that grows as your garden grows. Income that gives you opportunities.

Because here's what most people don't realize: the knowledge you've gained from this book, the plants you're growing, the systems you're building, and the monetary value you earn.

People will pay for what you know. They'll pay for what you grow. They'll pay for your time, your expertise, your plants, and your produce.

You just have to know how to package it, where to sell it, and how to do it legally and sustainably.

Let me show you how.

Start with what you have (right now)

Don't wait until you have acres of land, or a perfect Instagram feed, or a greenhouse full of exotic plants.

Start with what you have right now. Today.

Look around your property and ask yourself:

Do you have plants you can propagate? Lemongrass clumps you can divide? Moringa cuttings? Aloe pups? Katuk branches that root easily?

Do you have extra fruit you're not using? Mangoes, papayas, guavas, bananas that would otherwise rot or go to the birds?

Do you have knowledge that beginners would pay for? Can you teach someone how to plant their first fruit tree? How to start a small herb garden? How to grow food in Florida's heat?

Do you have compost, mulch, or worm castings?

That's your starting inventory. And every single one of those things can generate income.

Money grows when you start small and reinvest in better tools, more seeds, and expanded systems.

You don't need to launch a full business tomorrow. You just need to make your first $20. Then your first $100. Then build from there.

Sell What You Grow (Legally)

Depending on your area, you can sell produce, seeds, cuttings, or starter plants.

Let me be clear: you need to check your local laws and regulations. Some counties require permits for selling food. Some cities have cottage food laws that allow small-scale sales. Inspections or certifications are required by some farmers' markets.

Do your homework. Talk to your local agricultural extension office. Join local gardening groups and ask what others are doing.

But once you know the rules, here's what sells well in Florida:

Tropical plants: Moringa seedlings, passion fruit vines, Barbados cherry cuttings, banana pups, lemongrass divisions. These are in demand year-round in zones 9-11.

Culinary herbs: fresh basil, cilantro, parsley, mint, Thai basil, lemongrass stalks. Restaurants and home cooks will buy these weekly if the quality is good.

Medicinal herbs: Dried moringa, turmeric root, ginger, aloe vera plants, katuk cuttings. The wellness crowd pays premium prices for fresh, local, organically grown medicinal plants.

Specialty produce: Things grocery stores don't carry. Seminole pumpkins, passion fruit, guava, Barbados cherries, sugar cane, fresh turmeric.

Seeds and cuttings: People want to grow their own. Sell what propagates easily.

Pro tip: Bundle products.

A "Beginner's Florida Herb Garden" with three starter plants sells better than three individual plants.

A "Medicinal Tea Garden Kit" with moringa, lemongrass, and ginger sells at a premium.

A "Tropical Fruit Tree Package" with care instructions adds value.

People pay more for convenience and confidence. Give them both.

Teach What You Know

If you've been growing food for even a year or two, you already know over 90% of people.

That knowledge has value.

You can turn it into income through:

Paid workshops: Host a 2-hour Saturday morning workshop in your backyard. "How to Start a Florida Food Forest." "Growing Medicinal Herbs in Zone 10." "Fruit Trees for Beginners." Charge $25 to $50 per person. Get 10 people;25 to $50 that's $250-500 for a morning's work.

Online courses: Record videos teaching what you know. Sell access on platforms like Teachable, Gumroad, or your own website. Create once, sell repeatedly.

Consulting: Charge by the hour to walk someone's property and create a planting plan. People will pay $100-200 for an hour of your time if you save them from making expensive mistakes.

E-books and guides: Write a simple PDF guide on a specific topic. "10 Easy Herbs for Florida Beginners." "The First-Year Food Forest Planting Schedule." Sell it for $7 to $15. It's passive income once it's created.

YouTube ad revenue: Consistent content on YouTube can generate $100-500+ per month once you're monetized (1,000 subscribers, 4,000 watch hours).

Here's the key: Beginners don't want everything you know. They want simple steps to get started without killing their plants.

Give them that. Make it clear, actionable, and encouraging. They'll pay for it.

Content Is Currency

In today's world, you can turn your journey into income if you're willing to document it.

I've done this with GrowFitFL on YouTube. I document what I'm doing anyway: planting, pruning, harvesting, training, and people watch. Some of those viewers end up as customers. Some people decide to become students. A few merely provide support for the channel.

But it all starts with showing up consistently and providing value.

Take photos. Film short videos. Share your mistakes and your wins. Show the process, not just the results.

Platforms like YouTube, TikTok, and Instagram can lead to:

Ad revenue: YouTube pays you based on views once you're monetized. It's not huge at first, but it compounds.

Sponsorship deals: Companies will pay you to feature their products if you have an engaged audience. Seeds, tools, soil amendments, anything related to gardening.

Affiliate commissions: Recommend products you actually use and earn a percentage when people buy through your link. Amazon Associates, specialized garden suppliers, tool companies.

Direct product sales: Use your platform to sell your own products, plants, guides, and courses.

But here's the truth: if you're not consistent, it won't grow.

You can't post three times and expect results. You can't disappear for months and expect people to stick around.

Treat content like a crop. Plant regularly. Water it with effort. Give it time.

I've been posting on YouTube for years. Some videos get 500 views. Some get 50,000. But I keep showing up. And over time, the audience grows. The income grows. The opportunities grow.

If you're willing to do the same, the platform is there waiting for you.

Partner With Local Businesses

Your plants, your produce, and your knowledge can be valuable to local businesses.

And working with businesses gives you consistent, reliable buyers instead of depending on random customers.

Here's what I've seen work:

Sell herbs to tea shops or health food stores: Fresh or dried moringa, lemongrass, ginger, turmeric. Build a relationship with the owner, deliver quality consistently, and you've got a recurring customer.

Supply tropical fruit to local juice bars or restaurants: passion fruit, guava, papaya, things they can't get from regular suppliers.

Grow specialty crops for chefs: High-end restaurants will pay premium prices for fresh, local, unusual produce. Talk to chefs. Ask what they can't find.

Provide starter plants to nurseries: If you can propagate reliably, nurseries might buy wholesale from you.

Teach workshops at garden centers: They have the space and the audience. You provide the expertise. Split the revenue.

Relationships matter here. Show up on time. Deliver what you promise. Communicate clearly.

Your reputation is everything in a small business. Protect it.

Diversify Your Income Streams

Never rely on one income source.

If all your income comes from selling plants and a freeze kills your inventory, you're stuck.

If all your income comes from YouTube and the algorithm changes, you're in trouble.

Diversification protects you.

You might start with plant sales. After that, add an e-book. Then, a monthly workshop. Next, affiliate links. Then a small course.

Over time, those streams add up.

Example monthly income (realistic, not inflated):

- Plant sales at farmers' market: $200
- YouTube ad revenue: $150
- One workshop per month: $300
- E-book sales: $75
- Affiliate commissions: $100

Total: $825/month doing what you love.

That's not quit-your-job money for most people. But it's grocery money. It's saving money. It's investment-in-the-garden money.

And it's proof that your knowledge and your work have real market value.

Plus, these numbers grow over time as you refine your systems, expand your audience, and improve your products.

Keep it legal and sustainable

This is important: do it right.

Check local laws: Research what you're allowed to sell in your area. Cottage food laws vary by state and county. Some places require permits, licenses, or inspections.

Keep records for taxes: Even side hustle income is taxable. Keep receipts, track expenses, and report income. Don't give the IRS a reason to come knocking.

Don't burn yourself out: The fastest way to kill your love for gardening is to turn it into a stressful, all-consuming job. Build systems so your side hustle works with your life, not against it.

Maintain quality: what you deliver builds your reputation. Don't sell inferior products just to make a quick buck. People remember.

Price fairly: Don't undervalue your work, but don't price yourself out of the market either. Research what others are charging and price higher. Competing on price is a losing strategy; sell quality and give great customer service. You can have 1000 customer paying a little or 100; pricing will be higher for the 100 customers as the goal will be to earn as much as the 1000 customers.

Start small, scale slowly: test one income stream at a time. Get good at it. Then add another. Trying to do everything at once is a recipe for failure.

Your garden can feed you in many ways

Your garden feeds you with food. That's the foundation.

But it can also feed you with income, purpose, community, and skills that translate to dollars.

Start with what you know. Grow into what you don't. Let your skills put money back in your pocket.

A side hustle isn't just extra cash. It's proof that your knowledge, your hands, and your hard work have real value.

It's proof that you don't have to depend entirely on a paycheck from someone else.

It's proof that the things you love, the things you'd do anyway, can also subsidise you.

That's a different harvest. And it's worth pursuing.

So look at what you've built. What you're growing. What you know.

There's income there if you're willing to see it and willing to do the work to monetize it.

Start small. Stay legal. Build slowly. Reinvest. Diversify.

And watch what grows.

Not just in your garden. But in your bank account. In your options. In your freedom.

That's the goal. That's the opportunity.

Now make it happen.

Chapter 17

THE GARDEN AFTER YOU

One day, your hands won't turn this soil anymore.

Someone else will.

That thought used to bother me. Now it drives me harder than anything else.

Because the truth is simple.

A garden doesn't end when you do.

When I plant a mango tree, I already understand what I'm signing up for. It will take years to reach its full strength. I'll get fruit, sure. But the best harvest will belong to someone else.

Maybe my kids.

Maybe my grandkids.

Maybe a stranger.

Maybe a child who hasn't even been born yet.

And that's the beauty of it.

I'm not just planting into dirt. I'm planting for the future.

Think about the old homesteads you've seen. Pecan trees keep dropping. The fig trees still stand guard. The citrus still feeds whoever shows up when the season is right.

The original gardener is long gone.

But their work is still doing its job.

That's a legacy no politician can erase. No market crash can wipe out. No storm can fully destroy.

We live in a world obsessed with speed. Buy it now. Fix it fast. Replace it. Move on.

Gardens refuse to play that game.

They move at a different rhythm.

They stretch slow. They root deep. And in that patience, they remind us of what actually lasts.

The avocado you plant this spring could one day shade your grandchildren's backyard cookouts.

The lemon tree you prune today could still teach patience fifty years from now.

That's what I mean by The Garden After You.

It's not just food.

It's a story.

It's your hands still working long after they're gone. It's proof you were here. Proof you cared enough to build something meant to outlive your own breath.

So plant boldly.

Write your name in the ground, not on a plaque.

Let your garden speak for you when you no longer can.

Let it feed the hungry.

Let it shade the weary.

Let it remind whoever comes next that someone before them believed life was worth cultivating.

Because one day the tomatoes will rot.
The weeds will creep back in.
The tools will rust.
But that tree will still stand.
Roots sunk deep.
Fruit in season.
Quietly telling the world that you didn't just exist.
You grew.

And long after the house changes hands, after the fence falls and gets rebuilt, after the memories fade and the stories blur, that tree will still be there.

Still giving.
Still holding the shape of your decision to care.
That is how you stay.
Not in words.
Not in titles.
Not in things that disappear.
But in living systems that keep going.
That is the garden after you.

Chapter 18

THE CALL TO ACTION

If you've made it this far, you already know what's at stake.

They did not build the system for you. The creators designed it to keep you dependent. To keep you buying, consuming, working, and never quite getting ahead.

The hidden costs are bleeding you dry while your health, your time, and your family slip through your fingers.

You've seen it with your own eyes.

Shelves empty overnight. Prices are climbing every month. Bodies breaking down from processed food and sedentary living. Kids are getting sicker, weaker, more dependent.

And somewhere deep inside, you knew it didn't have to be this way.

That's why you picked up this book.

To shake you out of the comfortable numbness that keeps you scrolling instead of planting. Buying instead of building. Hoping instead of acting.

Because hope without action is just dreaming. And dreaming doesn't feed your family.

Here's what you've learned

Your health is a garden. If you don't plant it, tend it, and protect it, someone else will profit from selling you pill, procedures, and processed food. Your body wants to heal. You just have to give it the tools.

Resilience isn't theory. You rarely read about or discuss it. It's putting roots in the dirt and strength in your body. It's building systems that work when everything else fails.

You start where you are, with what you've got, or you stay stuck. There's no perfect time. No perfect place. No perfect plan. There's only now. And what you do with it.

You can eat every single month of the year if you know what to grow. Cool-season, warm season, perennials that produce year-round. The blueprint is right here. You don't need a farm. You need courage to begin.

The herbs under your feet are medicine. Moringa, lemongrass, ginger, turmeric, aloe. Either you learn them, grow them, and use them, or you keep paying for someone else's solutions while your health deteriorates.

Time and money are not excuses. They are resources. And you control where they go. You can spend them on Netflix and takeout, or you can invest them in a food forest that feeds you for decades. That's a choice.

Training your body is non-negotiable. A weak body can't protect your family. Can't build your garden. Can't endure the storms. Strength isn't vanity. It's survival. It's stewardship of the one body you'll ever have.

A fortress home means a garden to feed you, a gym to strengthen you, and a library to sharpen you. Miss one, and you're exposed. These three elements combine to create a life that is secure from being taken away.

Your kids are watching. Everything you do, they absorb. What you plant, they inherit. Weakness or resilience. Dependence or freedom. Excuses or action. That choice is yours, and it echoes through generations.

And when you're gone, the garden will speak louder than your words ever could. The trees you planted will feed people you'll never meet. The systems you built will provide long after your voice fades. That's a legacy.

Stripped Down to the Essentials

So here it is, stripped down to what matters:

Either you plant, or you remain a prisoner.

A prisoner of grocery stores that control what you eat.

A prisoner to pharmaceutical companies that profit from your sickness.

A prisoner to a system that wants you weak, distracted, and dependent.

You don't need permission to break free. You don't need the perfect spot, the perfect tools, or a college degree in soil science.

You need grit.

You need to step outside, put a seed in the ground, and water it.

Not tomorrow. Not when life slows down. Not when you have more money, or more time, or more certainty.

Today.

Right now.

Because a year from now, you'll either be walking through your own garden, feeding your family with food you grew, standing under trees you planted, harvesting herbs that heal your body…

Or you'll be exactly where you are right now, wishing you had started.

Older. More tired. Still dependent. Still waiting.

And that year will have passed either way.

The only difference is what you choose to do with it.

This Isn't Just About Food

This isn't just about tomatoes, or mangoes, or sweet potatoes.

This is about food freedom.

About being untouchable when the shelves are empty. In the event of a power outage. As the storms move in. When prices spike. When supply chains break.

It's about building something no one can take from you.

Not the government. Not the economy. Not the chaos of the world.

Your food. Your strength. Your knowledge. Your legacy.

Those are yours. And once you build them, they're unshakeable.

That's what this book has been about from the beginning.

Not gardening tips, or fitness advice, or random information.

But a complete system for building a life that external forces. Can't break.

A life rooted in something real.

Your Final Assignment

So here's your final assignment. The only one that matters.

Close this book.

Put it down.

Go outside.

Put your hands in the soil.

Plant something.

It doesn't have to be big. It doesn't have to be perfect.

A single moringa seed. One sweet potato slip. One lemongrass division.

Just plant something that will outlive your excuses.

Plant something that will feed your family.

Plant something that will shout to the world: I took control.

And then tomorrow, do it again.

Water that seed. Plant another one. Move your body. Read something that makes you sharper.

Establish the habit. Build the system. Build the life.

One day at a time. One plant at a time. One workout at a time.

Because this is how freedom develops. Not in grand gestures, but in daily disciplines that compound.

The time for reading is over

You've read enough.

You understand the necessary actions. You know why it matters. You know what's at stake.

The time for reading is over.

The time for planning is over.

The time for waiting for the perfect moment is over.

The time for planting is now.

So put this book on your shelf. Let it be a reference when you need it.

But don't let it be an excuse to delay.

Don't let knowledge replace action.

Don't let inspiration fade into procrastination.

Go. Now. Today.

Plant.

Train.

Build.

Learn.

And in a year, when you're harvesting fruit from trees you planted, when you're stronger than you've been in decades, when your kids are eating food they helped grow, when you feel truly free for the first time in your life...

Remember this moment.

The moment you started.

The moment you decided to become independent.

The moment you took control.
That's the moment everything changed.
And it starts now.
See you in the garden.
- Jermaine
GrowFitFL

Chapter 19

WINTER PROTECTION

How to protect fruit trees and gardens when Florida pretends it's the Arctic

I wish this chapter didn't need to exist. But here we are.

The winter of 2026 has been brutal. Not the coldest headline or the most dramatic social media clip. I mean the cold that hangs around long enough to actually kill things. Multiple nights below freezing. Real stress on tropicals. The damage that makes you question what you planted and where.

I'm not trying to predict the future. Nobody knows if we'll see winters like this again. But I know this much. If it happens again, I want you ready. A food forest is an investment. Time, money, years of growth. Winter protection is how you keep all that from disappearing in one awful week.

This chapter walks you through the entire plan. Preparation, emergency moves, recovery. I'll give you the standard stuff everyone talks about, and I'll also show you the tactics that separate hoping your trees survive from actually keeping them alive.

Important safety note

Don't risk your life, your family, or your home to save a plant. Cold protection should never create a fire hazard or carbon monoxide risk. If something involves flame, fuel, or electricity, use common sense and keep a safe distance. If you're not sure, skip it.

Step 1: Know what you're fighting

Cold damage isn't just one thing.

Frost forms on surfaces when temperatures drop, and the surface cools below freezing. You can get frost even when the air reads above 32 degrees.

A freeze happens when air temperatures hit 32 or below and plant tissue actually freezes inside.

Wind makes everything worse. Arctic winds pull heat off leaves and branches fast. It can turn a light cold snap into serious damage.

How long it lasts matters more than the coldest number. One quick dip overnight? Your plants can probably handle it. Two or three nights in a row? That's when tropical trees start dying back.

Step 2: Rank your plants by risk today

Before the cold hits, you need a plan. Every yard has limited time and limited supplies.

Make three lists.

Red list: protect at all costs

Newly planted trees

Anything in a pot

Tropicals, especially under 3 years old

Any tree you can't replace easily, whether it's expensive or sentimental

Anything flowering or holding fruit that you actually want

Yellow list: protect if you have time

Established tropicals with some size on them

Plants already under a canopy or near the house

Green list: they'll be fine

Cold tolerant citrus

Hardy established trees in warm spots

Anything you can replace without crying about it

This keeps you from burning energy on your toughest plants while your fragile ones freeze.

Step 3: Build your kit before you need it

Wait until the cold front is here and you'll overpay for stuff that doesn't work.

Here's what actually matters.

Frost cloth

Not a bedsheet. Not plastic. Real frost cloth breathes and holds warmth without trapping moisture that'll freeze.

Clamps and stakes

You need to pin the fabric to the ground. Heat escapes from the bottom first.

Mulch

Wood chips, leaves, straw, whatever insulates soil. Bare dirt loses heat like crazy.

Old-school **incandescent Christmas lights**

Not LEDs. LEDs put out no heat. Incandescent strings add warmth under a cover.

Buckets, trash cans, storage totes

For small trees and sensitive plants, hard covers work better than you'd think.

Water source and hose

For managing soil moisture and last-minute options.

Thermometer you actually trust

Get one that records the low temperature. Put it in the coldest part of your yard so you're not guessing.

Step 4: Win the microclimate game

Most people lose plants because they treat their whole yard the same way . Your yard has warm spots and cold spots.

Warm zones

South and west sides of the house

Near block walls, fences, patios, concrete

Under canopy trees that hold heat

Near water, even small ponds

Cold zones

Low spots where cold air settles

Open windy areas

The middle of the yard, away from anything

Anywhere with a clear sky overhead and no cover

If you can move pots, do it now. Push them against the house, under an overhang, pack them together. Grouping them tightly cuts down heat loss. Easiest win you'll get.

Step 5: Water the right way, at the right time

People get worked up about this. Don't. It's just physics.

Wet soil holds and releases heat better than dry soil. You want the root zone moist before the cold arrives.

What to do?

Water the day before the coldest night, in the afternoon, so the soil has time to soak it up and store heat.

What not to do

Don't drench everything late at night and leave it soaking wet if temps are going to stay below freezing for hours. You'll just make ice. And don't think overhead watering is always safe. It can help in specific situations if you do it right, but mess it up and you'll cause more damage. Stick with soil moisture, covers, and wind protection.

Step 6: Cover like you mean it

Covering isn't about hiding the plant. It's about trapping heat from the ground.

The rules

Your cover has to reach the ground. If it's floating above the soil, you're not trapping anything.

Use stakes or a frame so the cloth doesn't crush tender growth.

Clamp it tight at the bottom so the wind doesn't blow cold air inside.

Double layer for really sensitive plants.

If it's windy, put up a windbreak first, then cover.

What people screw up

Plastic touching leaves. Plastic conducts cold and will freeze leaf tissue on contact. If you use plastic, it goes over a frame, never touching the plant, and you have to vent it or take it off during the day.

Sheets and towels. They soak up water, get heavy, and collapse. You can use them in a pinch, but frost cloth is way better.

Step 7: Add heat, but do it safely

When the forecast looks nasty, covers alone might not cut it, especially for young tropicals.

Heating **options that won't burn your house down**

Incandescent Christmas lights under frost cloth

Wrap them loose around the trunk and inner branches, then cover everything to the ground. This can bump the temperature slowly inside the cover a few degrees, which is usually the difference between leaf burn and serious dieback.

Warm water jugs

Fill gallon jugs or dark buckets with warm water and set them under the cover near the trunk, not touching it. They release heat slow all night.

Compost heat

A compost pile near sensitive plants creates a warmer zone. Even an enormous pile of fresh mulch helps, especially if the plant is on the warm side of it.

Big tote method for small trees

If the tree's still small enough, drop a storage tote or trash can over it late afternoon. Toss a jug of warm water inside. Pull it off in the morning when the temps come up. Works better than you'd expect.

What I don't recommend

Open flames near cloth, gas heaters, charcoal, anything that makes carbon monoxide or starts fires. If you know what you're doing and have a safe setup, fine. If not, don't learn this lesson the hard way.

Step 8: Protect the trunk, because the trunk is the tree

Leaves grow back. A dead trunk ends everything.

For young tropical trees, trunk protection is huge.

Wrap frost cloth around the trunk

Add foam pipe insulation to the lower trunk of really young trees

Mulch heavy around the base, but don't pile it against the trunk

If you have to pick between covering the canopy or protecting the trunk, protect the trunk

Step 9: Emergency moves when the forecast worsens

Sometimes the forecast changes and you're out of time. Here's what you do.

Potted plants

Shove them against the house, pack them close, cover the entire group like one big unit.

Small in ground trees

Use the tote method. Or throw up a quick frame with stakes and wrap frost cloth around it to the ground.

Medium trees

Double-layer frost cloth, add incandescent lights, seal the bottom, throw up a windbreak on the north and west sides.

Large established trees

Focus on the trunk and lower branches. Heavy mulch. Lights on the trunk, if you can manage it. Windbreaks were possible. You're not wrapping a 15-foot tree, so protect what matters most.

Real talk

In bad cold snaps, some tropicals are going to take damage, anyway. You're not aiming for perfection. You're aiming for survival and a faster comeback.

Step 10: The morning after

This is where people mess up and turn damage they could recover from into permanent damage.

Don't prune right away

Wait until the weather settles. Damaged leaves still protect branches from the sun and more cold. Prune too early, and you expose tender tissue and invite disease.

Vent covers when the sun comes out

If temps rise during the day, crack open your covers so you don't cook your plants.

Water normal, don't flood

Keep your usual routine. Stressed roots hate extremes.

Check the trunk

If you see splits, oozing, soft spots, leave it alone and give it time. Shade it from the sun if you need to.

Step 11: Recovery after the cold wave

Once the cold breaks, you shift from defense to rebuilding.

Wait to prune until **you see** fresh growth

Fresh growth shows you what's alive. Only prune back to living wood.

Feed light, not heavily

A stressed tree doesn't need a fertilizer bomb. Start gently with compost, build up later.

Shade if needed

After cold damage, bright sun can fry weakened tissue. Temporary shade cloth helps.

Write about what happened

Note which plants struggled and where. That's how you design a smarter garden. Most people repeat the same mistakes because they never track what went wrong.

Tactics that actually work

Design for protection

Plant tropical trees in the open, and they'll always be vulnerable.

Clustering them, layering the canopy, buffering the wind. That's not just pretty. That's armor.

Use nurse plants

Fast-growing plants create windbreaks and warm pockets for slower tropicals. Even temporary shrubs help.

Mound for drainage, mulch for heat

Stressed roots worsen cold damage. A tree sitting wet and cold is getting hit twice. Good planting and drainage protect your trees long before winter shows up.

Build a winter corner

Pick one side of your yard as your winter refuge. Near the house. Near walls. With power access to the lights. This becomes your go-to zone for pots and high-value plants.

Last word

I can't promise Florida won't hit us with another winter like 2026. Nobody can. What I can promise is this. Being ready changes what happens.

A protected garden keeps paying you back. Fruit. Health. Lower grocery bills. Peace of mind.

Take one thing from this chapter; take this. Don't wait until the first frost warning to get serious. What you do before winter decides what you still have after winter.

Chapter 20

RECOVERY AFTER DISASTER

How to rebuild when Florida hits back

If you garden in Florida long enough, something's going to hit you.

Hard freeze. Hurricane. Weeks of rain drowning roots. Drought cracking the soil. Or maybe life gets heavy, and the garden sits there longer than you meant it to.

This chapter isn't about stopping disasters. It's about what you do afterwards.

Most books talk about prevention and stop there. Almost none tell you how to actually recover. That's a problem because recovery is where most people walk away for good.

I've been through all of it. Freezes that blackened entire trees overnight. Storms that snapped branches I thought were untouchable. Stretches where I couldn't keep up and had to watch things suffer. Every time I learned something that made the next recovery faster.

This chapter gives you what I learned the hard way so you don't have to.

The first rule after any disaster

Do nothing immediately.

Sounds backwards. It's not.

After extreme stress, plants need time to show you what actually survived. Cutting too fast, digging too soon, and trying to fix everything immediately usually does more damage than the disaster itself.

Your job at first is to watch and wait.

Cold damage recovery

After a freeze, plants look worse than they are. Leaves turn black. Stems look lifeless. Fruit drops everywhere. This is normal panic from the plant, not necessarily death.

What to leave alone

Any plant with green under the bark

Any branch that bends instead of snapping clean

Any trunk that's still firm, even if the top looks trashed

What not to do

Don't prune right away

Don't hit it with fertilizer

Don't assume it's dead because it looks ugly

Here's why. Those dead-looking leaves? They're actually protecting living tissue underneath from sunburn and more cold if another front rolls through. Rip them off too early and you expose tender branches that can't handle it yet.

Wait till temps settle and stay warm. When you see fresh growth pushing out somewhere, anywhere, that's your green light. I typically give my trees 3-6 weeks of doing nothing to them after a freeze.

When to cut after cold

Once fresh growth appears, prune back to living wood only. Make clean cuts with sharp tools. Cut into a branch and see green or wet tissue? Stop right there. Brown and dry all the way through? Go back further until you hit living wood.

If the whole top is dead but the trunk is alive, the tree can still come back. It won't look the same for a year or two, but it's not lost. I've had mango trees come back from stumps. Took three years to fruit again, but they made it.

One thing nobody tells you. Sometimes the main trunk dies, but the rootstock below the graft survives and sends up shoots. You'll get growth, but it won't be the variety you planted. Decide if you want to keep it or start over. I've kept a few just to have the shade and structure while I replant nearby.

Hurricane and wind damage recovery

Wind doesn't break things cleanly. Trees split, twist, tear. Roots half pull up. It's messy.

Priority

Safety. Get rid of anything that can fall on someone. Forget about shaping or making it pretty. That comes later.

What to remove immediately

Broken limbs hanging or split partway

Branches with torn bark that can't heal

Trees completely uprooted that you can't reset in the next day or two

What to leave?

Leaning trees with root balls still mostly in the ground

Trees that lost leaves but whose structure is intact

Trees that look stripped bare but nothing snapped

A lot of trees that look destroyed after a hurricane will push out new leaves within a month. Windburn and leaf loss aren't death sentences. I've seen trees look like sticks in September and have full canopies by December.

If a tree is leaning but the roots are holding, you can stake it temporarily. Don't leave the stake on forever. Once it anchors again, pull the stake. Trees that move a little in the wind rebuild stronger root systems than ones tied rigidly.

What actually kills trees after hurricanes

Salt spray if you're near the coast. It burns leaves and can poison soil if it's heavy enough. If you get hit with salt spray, hose down everything you can reach as soon as it's safe. A freshwater rinse makes a difference.

Root damage you can't see. A tree might look fine above ground, but half the roots tore when it shifted. Those trees decline slowly over months. There's not much you can do except water them steadily and hope they reRoot before they give up.

Flooding recovery

Flooding is one of the quietest killers in Florida. Roots drown, and by the time you see the damage, it's often too late to fix.

Signs of flood stress

Leaves yellowing days or weeks after the water goes down

Sudden leaf drop when nothing else changed

Soil smells sour or rotten

Roots are soft, dark, or slimy if you dig down to check

What to do?

Don't fertilize. Damaged roots can't take up nutrients, and you'll just burn what's left.

Improve drainage as soon as the ground firms up enough to work.

Pull back the mulch temporarily if the ground remains soggy. Let it breathe.

Give it time. Some trees bounce back once oxygen gets back to the roots. Others decline slow.

Flood damage shows up late. A tree can look fine for a month, then suddenly collapse. That's because the roots rotted underwater and it took that long for the tree to run out of reserves.

What survives flooding better than you'd think
Bald cypress (obviously, it's a swamp tree)
Mulberry
Elderberry
Taro and other wetland crops
Some citrus on the right rootstock

What rarely makes **it**
Avocado (root rot city)
Most tropical fruit trees, if flooded for more than a few days,
Anything already stressed before the flood

If you're in a flood-prone area, design for it. Plant on mounds. Use swales to move water away from tree roots. Pick species that tolerate wet feet. I learned this one the expensive way.

Drought recovery

Drought sneaks up on you. Plants look okay, then one day they're not.

What bounces back well?
Established trees with deep roots
Native plants or anything adapted to Florida for years
Anything growing in heavily mulched soil

What struggles?

Young trees without established roots

Shallow rooted vegetables

Anything growing in straight sand with no organic matter

After a drought, don't flood everything all at once. Dry soil, especially sandy soil, can repel water at first. It'll run right off instead of soaking in. Water deep and slow. Let it soak. Come back and water again.

Mulch makes the biggest difference here. I've seen the same species planted ten feet apart. One mulched, one bare soil. The mulched one sailed through a dry spell. The other one fried in the sun. It's that simple.

Neglect recovery

This one's harder to talk about, but it's real.

Sometimes life happens. You get busy. Someone gets sick. Work explodes. You miss weeks, maybe months. The garden sits there and suffers.

The good news? Plants want to live. Most of them will hang on longer than you think.

Start simple

Water consistently, even if nothing else gets done

Pull out the obvious dead stuff so you can see what's left

Add mulch to help everything hang on

Don't catch up with heavy fertilizer. You'll stress weak plants worse.

A lot of plants rebound fast once basic care returns. Some won't. That's okay. You're not a poor gardener because life got in the way.

I've had stretches where I couldn't keep up. Garden looked rough. I felt terrible about it. But once I got back to basics, most things came back. The ones that didn't? I replaced them and moved on.

How to tell what's actually dead

Scratch the bark lightly with your thumbnail. Green underneath means it's alive. Brown and dry means it's dead at that spot. Keep checking lower until you find green or hit the ground.

Check the base of the trunk. If it's soft, caving in, or smells rotten, the tree's done. No coming back from trunk rot.

Look for fresh growth at the base or along the trunk. Even if the top is completely dead, shoots from the base mean the roots are still alive and trying.

Dead wood doesn't come back. But living roots can surprise you six months later.

What rebounds better than people expect

Moringa. You can cut it to the ground, and it'll shoot back up.

Cassava. Nearly indestructible.

Sweet potato. The vines might die, but the tubers usually survive and re-sprout.

Banana. Cut down to nothing, and it sends up pups from the rhizome.

Mulberry. Tough as nails. I've seen them come back from stumps.

Pigeon pea. Handles drought, handles neglect, keeps going.

Citrus. A lot of varieties will re-sprout from the trunk if the roots are healthy.

Tropical fruit trees, if the trunk survives the hit.

What rarely comes **back**

Trees with repeated root rot issues

Plants that had already been struggling for years before the disaster

Species planted way outside their comfort zone, trying to prove a point

Designing for faster recovery next time

Every disaster teaches you something if you pay attention.

Walk your yard after things settle. Observe the location where water accumulated. See which plants coped with the stress. Notice which spots stayed warmer, drier, or more protected. Notice what bounced back with almost no help.

Write it down. I'm serious. You'll forget otherwise.

Use that information to redesign. Move plants that struggled. Change spacing. Add drainage where water sat. Build berms or swales. Add windbreaks. Build up your soil so it holds moisture better or drains faster, depending on what you need.

A garden that survives disaster isn't lucky. It's designed by someone who paid attention to what went wrong last time.

I've moved trees three times before finding the right spot. Annoying? Yeah. But now they thrive instead of just surviving.

Closing thought

Disasters are going to happen. That doesn't mean your garden failed. That doesn't mean you failed.

Recovery is part of the deal. The gardeners who make it long-term aren't the ones who avoid loss. They're the ones who know how to rebuild without quitting.

I've lost trees I cared about. Plants I spent years growing. It hurt. But I learned from every single loss, and the garden I have now is stronger because of it.

This chapter exists so that one terrible season doesn't end your growing journey. You can come back from almost anything if you give it time and don't panic.

Chapter 21

WHY DO I GROW?

I started this whole thing because I was tired of watching my grocery bill climb while the quality of what I was buying dropped.

That's the truth. No grand mission. No deep philosophy. Just a dad looking at a receipt, thinking there has to be a better way to feed six people without going broke or filling them with garbage.

Twenty years later, I'm still out there every morning checking trees, pulling weeds, moving mulch. But the reasons have changed.

The money still matters. Don't get me wrong. Cutting our grocery bill in half freed up cash for things that matter. More trips to see a family in Ohio. Disney World without the guilt. Breathing room when unexpected expenses hit. That's real. That matters when you're raising four kids.

But somewhere along the way, something else happened.

I watched my kids grow up eating fruit they picked themselves. Not from a store. From a tree they helped plant. Having smelled hundreds of ripe mangoes, they are familiar with the scent. They can determine when a papaya is ripe. They know moringa leaves are edible and that sweet potatoes grow underground, not on trucks.

That knowledge doesn't come from a book or a screen. It comes from dirt under their fingernails and juice running down their chins.

My youngest, the one we had when we were in our 40s, he's known nothing different. For him, this is just how food works. You go outside and get it. I don't know if he will have a garden when he grows up. Maybe he won't. But he will always know it's possible. He will always know you don't have to depend on a system that doesn't care about you.

That matters more to me than I can put into words.

My wife, Toni, and I talk about this sometimes. About what we're really building here. This is more than just a garden. It's a different way of thinking. It's showing our kids that you don't have to accept what you're given. You can make something better with your own hands.

We still eat when the power goes out. When prices spike, we barely notice. When the world feels unstable, we walk outside and see the abundance we have created. That peace of mind, you can't buy that.

I've had people tell me they don't have time to garden. I get it. I'm busy too. Full schedule. Four kids. Making videos. Running a business. Trying to be present for my family. But here's what I learned. You make time for what matters. And this matters.

Because it's not just about the food.

It's about being outside instead of on a screen. It's about teaching your kids that hard work creates actual results. Knowing your neighbors is beneficial, especially when you have surplus fruit you can't consume quickly enough to give away. It's about building something that gets better every year instead of more expensive.

Building a YouTube channel or writing books was never my intention. I just wanted to help people avoid the mistakes I made. I wasted years doing things wrong. Planting in the wrong spot. Fighting my soil instead of working with it. Buying plants that had no business being in Florida.

If I can save you even one of those mistakes, this book has done its job.

But more than that, I hope this book gives you permission to start messy. To plant something and see what happens. It's about failing a bit and continuing regardless until you figure it out. Creating something to support your family, regardless of its appearance compared to Instagram photos.

Because most of my garden doesn't look perfect. It's productive. It's healthy. But it's not a showpiece. And that's fine. I'd rather eat well than photograph well.

Twenty years in, I'm still learning. Still making mistakes. Still adjusting. The garden teaches me something new every season, and I'm better for it.

What I want you to take from this book isn't just how to grow food. It's that you can. Right now. Where you are. With what you have.

You don't need perfect soil or perfect weather, or perfect timing. You need to start. Plant something. Water it. Learn from it. Build on it.

And one day, maybe not this year or next year, but one day, you'll walk outside and realize you're not worried about the grocery store anymore. You'll realize your kids know things most other kids don't. You'll realize you've built something that makes your life genuinely better.

That's what this gave me. That's what I hope it gives you.

Not perfection. Not a magazine spread. Just actual organic food, real savings, and real peace of mind.

Everything else is extra.

Jermaine Jefferson

West Central Florida, February 2026

Closing Words

AUTHOR'S NOTE

No one intended this book to serve as the last word.

It's the spark.

A spark to show you what's possible when you decide to take control of your food, your health, and your space.

My goal was simple: to share my journey in a way that gives you a simple starting point, practical ideas, and the motivation to take that first step.

Everything you've read here comes from my personal experience, the lessons I've learned, the mistakes I've made, and the systems that work for me and my family in West Central Florida.

It's not a one-size-fits-all formula.

Your climate might be different. Your budget, your time, your space, your needs, they'll all shape your unique path.

Take what makes sense for you. Leave what doesn't. Adapt everything to your own reality.

That's the beauty of this. There's no perfect way to do it. There's only your way, figured out through trial, error, and persistence.

If you want to go deeper, see these concepts in action, or connect with me directly, my YouTube channel, GrowFitFL, is where I share ongoing updates, tutorials, and real-life examples from my garden, my training, and my lifestyle.

You'll find:

- Step-by-step planting and pruning videos

- Live Q&As where I answer questions

- Garden tours showing what's actually working (and what's not)

- Workout demonstrations and training updates

- A community of people building their own systems, one seed at a time

This book is a guide. A foundation. A shortcut based on years of learning the hard way.

It's here to inspire you, shorten your learning curve, and help you avoid some mistakes I've made along the way.

But what do you do next? That's in your hands.

And that's the best part.

My permission is not required. You don't need to wait for more information. You have everything you need to start right now.

So go plant something.

Go build something.

Go live with the possibilities.

Praise God,

Jermaine

GrowFitFL

YouTube: @GrowFitFL

About The Author

Jermaine is the creator of GrowFitFL, a YouTube channel where gardening intersects with health, resilience, and real-life storytelling.

Based in West Central Florida, he teaches everyday people how to turn ordinary lawns into year-round food systems, grow medicinal and nutrient-dense plants, and build healthier, more self-sufficient lives regardless of space or experience level.

A husband, father of four, and lifelong student of natural living, Jermaine brings over twenty years of hands-on experience in gardening, fitness, and herbal research. His approach is practical, grounded, and designed for families dealing with actual conditions, not ideal scenarios.

GrowFitFL features step-by-step guidance, Florida-specific planting strategies, and honest conversations around food security, family, health, discipline, and legacy.

The content on GrowFitFL extends beyond the information in this book.

Behind the scenes, his food forest grows through the seasons, and you can watch plants move from seed to harvest in real time. You will learn not only how to grow food but also how to use it, from cooking with fresh herbs to preparing simple medicinal teas.

For those who want deeper access and ongoing support, Jermaine also shares exclusive content and community discussions through his GrowFitFL Patreon, created for readers and viewers who want to apply these lessons more intentionally.

You can learn more about Jermaine, his current projects, and the larger mission behind his work at jermainejefferson.com.

GrowFitFL is more than a channel. It is a growing community of people choosing to take responsibility for their health, their food, and their future, one seed at a time.

Follow GrowFitFL on YouTube to continue the journey.

Visit GrowFit.com to start your journey today

Jermaine lives in West Central Florida with his wife Toni and their four children, where he continues to expand his food forest, train daily, and share the journey with thousands of viewers around the world.

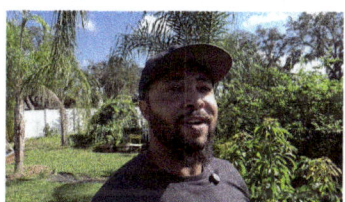

Jermaine Jefferson

Acknowledgments

Thank you for reading this book.

I didn't write it to impress anyone or just to hoping put my name on a cover. I wrote it to help.

Every page came from my own experiences, lessons learned the hard way, and a perspective I believe could make a difference in your life.

If even one idea here helps you grow your own food, improve your health, or see the world a little differently, then it's been worth every hour I spent creating it.

My goal was simple: to share what I've learned, hoping it might encourage, inspire, or equip you to act.

I truly appreciate the time you've given not just to read my words, but to consider them. Your willingness to listen means more to me than you know.

I hope this book leaves you with something valuable. Something you can carry forward and build on.

From my family to yours, thank you for letting me be a small part of your journey.

God bless you.

— Jermaine

Personal Thanks

To my wife, Toni: You've been my partner in every seed planted, every lesson learned, and every hard season weathered. This book exists because you believed in the vision before it had a name.

To my four children: You are the reason I plant trees I'll never climb. Everything in this book is for you, and for the future you'll build.

To my father: The roots you gave me run deeper than any tree I've planted. I carry your strength with me every day. I miss you.

To my mother: Your morning moringa tea and unwavering faith taught me that healing starts with what we choose to put in our bodies and our minds.

To the GrowFitFL community: Your questions, your stories, your commitment to building something real, you're the reason I keep showing up. This book is as much yours as it is mine.

To every person who's ever told me, "I wish I'd started sooner": This book is my answer. Start now. I'm with you.

And to God, my Lord and Savior: For provision, protection, and the wisdom to see that a garden is more than dirt and seeds. Praise God.

In Loving Memory of My Father

In loving memory of my father

"The greatest gift anyone could ever give me is to say that I remind them of my dad. His strength, his love, and his example live on through me."

www.ingramcontent.com/pod-product-compliance
Lightning Source LLC
Chambersburg PA
CBHW070612030426
42337CB00020B/3768